Lymph Node Surgery in Urology

Provided as a service to urology by

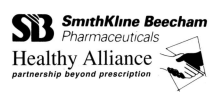

SB **SmithKline Beecham**
Pharmaceuticals

Healthy Alliance
partnership beyond prescription

Lymph Node Surgery in Urology

Edited by

John P. Donohue MD

Distinguished Professor Emeritus

Department of Urology,
University Hospital–1725,
Indiana University Medical Center,
550 N University Boulevard,
Indianapolis, Indiana 46202–5250, USA

I S I S
MEDICAL
MEDIA

Oxford

© 1995 by Isis Medical Media Ltd.
Saxon Beck, 58 St Aldates
Oxford, OX1 1ST, UK

First published 1995

British Library Cataloguing in Publication Data.
A catalogue record for this title is available from
the British Library

ISBN 1 899066 13 6

Donohue J.P. (John)
Lymph Node Surgery in Urology/
John P. Donohue

Always refer to the manufacturer's Prescribing
Information before prescribing drugs cited in this book.

Set by
Creative Associates, Oxford, UK

Printed by
Biddles Ltd.,
Guildford & Kings Lynn, UK

Distributed by
Times Mirror International Publishers
Customer Service Centre, Unit 1, 3 Sheldon Way,
Larkfield, Aylesford, Kent, ME20 6SF, UK

Contents

CONTENTS

List of Contributors

Carlos Allepuz Losa
Department of Urology, Hospital "Miguel Servet", via Isabel La Católica 1 and 3, 50009, Zaragoza, Spain

Jens E. Altwein MD
Professor of Urology, Urologist-in-Chief, Hospital Barmherzige Brueder, Romanstrasse 93, 80635 Munich, Germany

Yoshio Aso MD PhD FACS
Emeritus Professor, Department of Urology, Faculty of Medicine, University of Tokyo, 7-3-1 Hongo, Bunkyo-ku, Tokyo 113, Japan

Miguel Blas Marin
Department of Urology, Hospital "Miguel Servet", via Isabel La Católica 1 and 3, 50009, Zaragoza, Spain

Giorgia Carmignani MD
Professor of Urology, Chief of The Luciano Giuliani Institute of Urology, University of Genoa Medical School, S. Martino Hospital, viale Benedetto XV, I-16132 Genoa, Italy

Juan A. Casanova-Ramon MD
Consultant, Department of Urology, Instituto Valenciano de Oncología, C/- Prof. Beltran Baguena, 19, 46009 Valencia, Spain

James M. Cummings MD
Division of Urology, St. Louis University School of Medicine, 3635 Vista Avenue at Grand Boulevard, St. Louis, MO, 63110-0250, USA

Michele Cussotto MD
Resident, The Luciano Giuliani Institute of Urology, University of Genoa Medical School, S. Martino Hospital, viale Benedetto XV, I-16132 Genoa, Italy

Frans M. J. Debruyne MD PhD
Professor and Chairman, Department of Urology, University Hospital Nijmegen, Geert Grooteplein 16, P.O. Box 9101, 6500 HB Nijmegen, The Netherlands

LIST OF CONTRIBUTORS

Marian A. Devonec MD, PhD
Urology Department, Antiquaille Hospital, Lyon 69321, France

John P. Donohue MD
Department of Urology, University Hospital - 1725, Indiana University Medical Center, 550 N University Boulevard, Indianapolis, Indiana 46202-5250, USA

Robert E. Donohue MD
Professor of Surgery/Urology, University of Colorado Health Sciences Center, Division of Urology, 4200 East Ninth Avenue, Box C-319, Denver, CO, 80262, USA

Raimundo Dumont-Martinez MD
Consultant, Department of Urology, Instituto Valenciano de Oncología, C/- Prof. Beltran Baguena, 19, 46009 Valencia, Spain

Jean-Philippe Fendler MD
Assistant Professor in Urology, Hopital de l'Antiquaille, Université Claude Bernard, Lyon 1, France

Riccardo Franchini MD
Resident, The Luciano Giuliani Institute of Urology, University of Genoa Medical School, S. Martino Hospital, Genoa, Italy

Kimio Fujita MD PhD
Professor, Department of Urology, School of Medicine, Hamamatsu University, 3600 Handacho, Hamamatsu, Japan 431-31

Claudio Giberti MD
Staff Urologist, The Luciano Giuliani Institute of Urology, University of Genoa Medical School, S. Martino Hospital, viale Benedetto XV, I-16132 Genoa, Italy

Luciano Giuliani MD [†]
Professor of Urology, Chief of the Urology Department, University of Genoa Medical School, S. Martino Hospital, viale Benedetto XV, I-16132 Genoa, Italy

Vincente Guillem-Porta MD
Head of Department of Medical Oncology, Instituto Valenciano de Oncología, C/- Prof. Beltran Baguena, 19, 46009 Valencia, Spain

Laurence M. Harewood BSc MB BS FRACS
Urologist, Department of Urology, The Royal Melbourne Hospital, 6/206 Albert Street, East Melbourne, VIC, 3002, Australia

[†] Deceased August 18, 1994

Sverker Hellsten MD
Assistant Professor, Department of Urology, Malmö General Hospital, Sweden

Inmaculada Iborra-Juan MD
*Consultant, Department of Urology, Instituto Valenciano de Oncología,
C/- Prof. Beltran Baguena, 19, 46009 Valencia, Spain*

Akira Ishikawa MD
*Assistant, Department of Urology, School of Medicine, Hamamatsu University,
Handacho, Hamamatsu 431-13, Japan*

John A. Johnsen MD
Consultant, Department of Urology, County Hospital, Karlskrona, Sweden

Shuji Kameyama MD PhD
*Assistant Professor, Department of Urology, Faculty of Medicine, University of
Tokyo, 7-3-1 Hongo, Bunkyo-ku, Tokyo 113, Japan*

Kazuki Kawabe MD PhD
*Professor, Department of Urology, Faculty of Medicine, University of Tokyo,
7-3-1 Hongo, Bunkyo-ku, Tokyo 113, Japan*

David Kirk DM FRCS
*Consultant Urologist, West Glasgow Hospitals University NHS Trust and Honorary
Professor, Department of Urology, Gartnavel General Hospital,1053 Great Western
Road, Glasgow, G12 0YN, UK*

Carlos A. Levi D'Ancona
*Assistant Professor, Division of Urology, University of Campinas Medical Center,
UNICAMP, São Paulo, Brazil*

Giuseppe Martorana MD
Professor of Urology, Department of Urology, University of Bologna, Bologna, Italy

Etienne Mazeman MD
*Professeur des Universités, Praticien Hospitalier, Chef de Service, Clinique
Urologique, CHU Lille, France*

Jose L. Monrós-Lliso MD
*Consultant, Department of Urology, Instituto Valenciano de Oncología,
C/- Prof. Beltran Baguena, 19, 46009 Valencia, Spain*

Peter F. A. Mulders MD PhD
*Senior Resident, Department of Urology, University Hospital Nijmegen, Geert
Grooteplein 16, P.O. Box 9101, 6500 HB Nijmegen, The Netherlands*

LIST OF CONTRIBUTORS

Nicola Nicolai MD
Division of Urology, Istituto Nazionale Tumori, Via Venezian 1, 20133 Milan, Italy

Yoshihisa Ohtawara MD
Assistant, Department of Urology, School of Medicine, Hamamatsu University, 3600 Handacho, Hamamatsu 431-13, Japan

Francesco Oneto MD
Staff Urologist, The Luciano Giuliani Institute of Urology, University of Genoa Medical School, S. Martino Hospital, viale Benedetto, I-16132 Genoa, Italy

Raul O. Parra MD FACS
Professor and Chairman of Urology, Division of Urology, St. Louis University, School of Medicine, 3635 Vista Avenue at Grand Boulevard, St. Louis, MO, 63110-0250, USA

Paul M. Perrin MD
Professor and Chairman, Department of Urology, Hopital de L'Antiquaille, 1 rue de l'Antiquaille, F-69321 Lyon, Cedex 05, France

Luigi Piva MD
Division of Urology, Istituto Nazionale Tumori, Via Venezian 1, 20133 Milan, Italy

Giorgio Pizzocaro MD
Contract Professor of Urology, Director, Division of Urology, Istituto Nazionale Tumori, Via Venezian 1, 20133 Milan, Italy

Jose V. Ricós-Torrent MD
Consultant, Department of Urology, Instituto Valenciano de Oncología, C/- Prof. Beltran Baguena, 19, 46009 Valencia, Spain

Carlos Rioja Sanz MD
Department of Urology, Hospital "Miguel Servet", via Isabel La Católica 1 and 3, 50009, Zaragoza, Spain

Luis A. Rioja Sanz MD
Department of Urology, Hospital "Miguel Servet", via Isabel La Católica 1 and 3, 50009, Zaragoza, Spain

Nelson Rodrigues Netto Jr. MD
Professor and Chairman, Division of Urology, University of Campinas Medical Center, UNICAMP, São Paulo, Brazil

Salvatore Rovida MD
Professor of Medical Statistcs and Biometry, Institute of Medical Statistics and Biometrics, University of Genoa, Genoa, Italy

Eduardo Solsona MD
*Head of Department, Department of Urology, Instituto Valenciano de Oncología,
C/- Prof. Beltran Baguena, 19, 46009 Valencia, Spain*

Kazuo Suzuki MD PhD
*Associate Professor, Department of Urology, School of Medicine, Hamamatsu
University, 3600 Handacho, Hamamatsu 431-13, Japan*

David A. Swanson MD
*Professor, Department of Urology, The University of Texas M.D. Anderson Cancer
Center, 1515 Holcombe Boulevard, Houston, TX, 77030, USA*

Atsushi Tajima MD PhD
*Associate Professor, Department of Urology, Faculty of Medicine, University of
Tokyo, 7-3-1 Hongo, Bunkyo-ku, Tokyo 113, Japan*

Tomomi Ushiyama MD PhD
*Assistant Professor, Department of Urology, School of Medicine, Hamamatsu
University, 3600 Handacho, Hamamatsu 431-13, Japan*

Henk G. van der Poel MD PhD
*Junior Resident, Department of Urology, University Hospital Nijmegen, Geert
Grooteplein 16, P.O. Box 9101, 6500 HB Nijmegen, The Netherlands*

Preface

In all of cancer surgery, there is a question concerning lymphadenectomy in addition to removing the primary tumor itself. The concept of regional dissection becomes a compelling consideration, given the fact that malignant tumor spreads by both lymphatic and vascular extension. Only by extended clinical experience, can we glean enough information to make practical recommendations.

Even with extensive experience, questions remain as we study tumors of each organ system about the wisdom and propriety of regional lymphadenectomy in the surgical management of tumors of each primary organ involved. Questions remain, such as 'is associated regional lymphadenectomy simply a *staging* procedure?' or 'does regional lymphadenectomy also confer *therapeutic* benefit?'

In each of these solid tumor systems involved in urologic cancer, there are legitimate points of controversy regarding these two questions. In renal cancer, for example, there are rather divergent views which are presented herein. While it is true that most long term data suggests hematogenous spread is the determining factor in post nephrectomy clinical failures, there is some evidence to suggest that accurate and thorough regional lymphadenectomy will confer therapeutic benefit as well. It is probably true that this therapeutic benefit is modest, all things considered; but only through excellent clinical work and critique which follows, can the reader appreciate the nuances of the discussion about staging benefit versus therapeutic benefit of regional lymph node dissection.

It is generally agreed that limited regional lymphadenectomy with prostatectomy is of practical staging value, but little or no therapeutic value. On the other hand, both penile and testis cancer have remarkable clinical evidence in support of therapeutic value of regional lymphadenectomy. This becomes all the more cogent in the treatment of testis cancer where we have the option of initial platinum based combination chemotherapy for advanced disease followed by postchemotherapy regional lymphadenectomy. Good arguments examining these points are pro-offered in the chapters on penile and testis cancer.

In one area there is general agreement. Regional lymphadenectomy has therapeutic benefits, *per se*, independent of other treatment variables, in testicular cancer and in penile cancer. That is to say, a thorough regional lymphadenectomy in patients found to be node positive will confer survival advantage ranging from the 50th to the 66th percentile in patients found to have limited nodal burden of disease. There are few other cancers whereby cure can be obtained in node positive patients with surgery alone. These two organ systems require a thorough and practical understanding of surgical anatomy and technique in the management of primary tumor.

Hopefully this volume is timely and of practical value to the reader. Each contributor has an authoritative grasp of the issues and hopefully they are presented clearly. My thanks to the Société Internationale d'Urologie and to Etienne Mazeman and Michael Marberger for bringing this subject as a major theme of the 1994 Congress; and thanks to John Harrison for bringing this into published reality.

John P. Donohue, M.D.
Distinguished Professor Emeritus
Indiana University Medical Center

Acknowledgements

The Société Internationale d'Urologie has rapidly grown into one of the largest and most effective organizations in organized urology. This recent growth spurt over the last decade is due in no small measure to the exceptional efforts and talent of Etienne Mazeman who was Secretary General and President in this time frame. He was able to interest leading urologists world wide to support the concept of a supranational teaching organization embodied in the framework of the SIU.

At the penultimate SIU Meeting in Seville, 1991, topics for the next meeting were selected by the Program Committee and then Secretary, Michael Marberger. One of the five major themes was 'lymph node surgery and urologic cancer'. A panel of experts was convened, each of whom has recognized authority in a particular area. This book is a distillation of the proceedings of that meeting as given by these authorities in Sydney, Australia in September, 1994. We are grateful for the expert assistance of John Harrison of Isis Medical Media Ltd in organizing the aforementioned six topics into six attractive volumes. Most of all I am grateful to the contributors themselves, each of whom completed their assignments in a timely fashion.

John P. Donohue, M.D.
Distinguished Professor Emeritus
Indiana University Medical Center

Introduction

Role of lymph node dissection in urological cancer surgery

1

J. P. Donohue

Introduction

The role of lymph node dissection in cancer surgery is of staging value and, in some systems, of therapeutic value as well. In fact, the impact of any surgery on survival in many types of cancer can be difficult to prove. Recent biostatistical reviews indicate that the absolute survival in most cases of urological cancer is not significantly affected by prior manipulation; however, such data are amassed from all patients, many of whom have advanced disease at presentation. All reviewers are agreed that there is a role for surgery in a subset of cancer patients who appear to have localized disease. The immediate question pertains to the efficacy of associated lymph node dissection as an adjunct to surgery for the primary tumour.

As a general rule, the extent of such surgery should be appropriate to the needs of the patient. The goals are removal of the primary tumour for cure and removal of the regional lymph nodes for both staging information and possible *therapeutic* benefit. With the exception of testicular and penile cancer, the therapeutic impact of associated lymph node dissection per se is difficult to prove.

In the following sections, each tumour system is considered in turn.

Adrenal cancer

In adrenal cancer, lymph node dissection is essentially the same as for renal cancer, discussed below. The metastatic pattern for large adrenal tumours is usually haematological and the primary organs affected are pulmonary and hepatic, reflecting haematogenous spread. Surgery for larger adrenal tumours includes an ipsilateral nephrectomy.

Renal cancer

The role and extent of lymphadenectomy in this subset is controversial. Most agree that it is appropriate to perform an ipsilateral lymph node dissection in the course of a radical nephrectomy. The efficacy of extended bilateral lymph node dissection in surgery for renal cell carcinoma is being actively studied. There are some suggestive data, all retrospective, that suggest extended interval to relapse and possible survival in some patients with stage B and stage C disease, who were found to have regional lymph node involvement.[1-4] Further review of these patients indicates that most had incidental involvement and few had multiple or massive nodal involvement.[3,5-7] Generally speaking, a radical nephrectomy is inappropriate in the face of obvious gross nodal disease. There are many anecdotal cases of long-term survivors with one or more bulky positive node(s). In the past decade, radical nephrectomy in the presence of bulky nodal or multiple distant metastases became one of the more abused procedures in urology. The rationale of spontaneous regression after nephrectomy in such cases has not stood up to scrutiny and cooperative group studies have also shown that infarction and/or nephrectomy after infarction does not relate to significant regression or disappearance of the metastasis or increased patient survival.[4,9] Today, a reasonable consensus supports the practice of ipsilateral lymphadenectomy in the course of radical nephrectomy. This actually facilitates the vascular component of the procedure and may serve to reduce morbidity related to bleeding.

Ureteral cancer

Ureteral cancer is not usually associated with a systematic lymph node dissection unless it is located in the pelvis and this is much the same template as that for a radical nephrectomy, i.e. regional and ipsilateral dissection only. Furthermore, a lower ureteral lesion may warrant an ipsilateral pelvic nodal clearance for staging only. As a general rule, invasive ureteral tumours have a poor prognosis and survival is predetermined by biological factors, which function independently of any adjunctive surgical dissection.[10,11]

Prostate cancer

A lymph node dissection is of value in staging only, but may also redirect therapy. Examples would be discontinuing a planned total prostatectomy in the presence of positive nodes, a decision to re-treat the primary with another form of local treatment, such as radiotherapy, or a decision to perform bilateral orchiectomy at the time of discovery of positive nodes (with or without coincident prostatectomy and with or without additional total hormonal control with luteinizing hormone releasing hormone agonist or antagonist). Thus, lymphadenectomy in prostate cancer does have major prognostic value and may also redirect a variety of therapeutic options.[12]

Currently, the rapidly expanding technology of laparoscopic surgery lends itself quite well to pelvic lymphadenectomy. Although the 'learning curve' requires additional time, there are some possible cost and risk benefits to the procedure. The prospect of subsequent perineal prostatectomy is also appealing to some. These features are discussed in subsequent chapters (8–11).

Penile cancer

This is an epidermoid cancer characterized by local growth and regional nodal spread. Even advanced disease remains regional rather than distant. This is, therefore, one of the few types of primary cancer in which patients with positive nodes can enjoy long-term survival after thorough regional lymphadenectomy. In addition, even when lymph nodes in the groin are grossly enlarged, after a suitable period of observation it is appropriate to carry out lymph node dissection in these patients. The alternative, of continued observation, will be greeted with an even more morbid sequence of events, including local skin breakdown, separation and tumour erosion into the femoral vessels creating acute haemorrhagic emergencies. Data for early versus delayed groin dissection have been reviewed elsewhere.[13,14] In addition, the role of coincident pelvic dissection is the subject of debate. Most agree, however, that if groin dissection is negative for tumour, pelvic dissection can be withheld, although an exception to this rule might be where there is a lesion of the glans penis or a question or urethral extension, which would possibly involve direct pelvic extension through pathways in the corpus spongiosium that connect directly with the true pelvis.[13–15] Special efforts have been made to reduce the morbidity of simpler templates of dissection, but inguinal lymph node dissection for penile cancer should be thorough and complete for good therapeutic results and in order to preclude local recurrence.

Bladder cancer

The role of lymphadenectomy, together with radical cystectomy, for invasive bladder cancer becomes more interesting in the light of recent reviews. Historically, about 20% of patients undergoing cystectomy for bladder cancer were found to be 5-year survivors following resection of bladder with local pelvic nodal involvement. More recently, Skinner[16] has shown that as many as one-third of patients can be discovered to have positive nodes yet enjoy a 5-year survival. This is probably associated with several factors, including the meticulous care taken, both in dissection and in the examination of the en bloc specimen by the surgical pathologists. Another factor may relate to patient selection for treatment. Aggressive pursuit of patients with invasive disease, which is appropriate in the absence of negative clinical staging for distant metastases, will yield a higher incidence of nodal disease in referral centres, where extended cancer surgery is more commonly applied to patients with a generally higher level of local disease.

In any case, it makes very good sense to include thorough dissection of the pelvic lymph nodes in the course of a radical cystectomy. In fact, this approach provides better vascular exposure and, therefore, better vascular control throughout the procedure. Not only will this provide better pathological staging but also, as noted above, as many as one-third of patients, even those with stage D_1 disease, can be expected to survive beyond 5 years. Yet another factor promoting increased survival in patients today, compared with historical controls, are such features as better preoperative clinical staging, better nutritional support before and after surgery, and the advent of more effective adjuvant and neoadjuvant chemotherapy programmes. All these should be associated with an even better short-term survival in stage D_1 transitional cell carcinoma of the bladder.

The impact of neoadjuvant chemotherapy programmes remains to be seen, particularly in terms of absolute survival. It has not yet been demonstrated that patients with metastatic disease will have any significant prolongation of absolute survival in real time. However, relapse-free intervals and clinical downstaging are already apparent in several important ongoing studies. In fact, such studies have revealed some interesting facets of the biology of the disease, such as the emergence of central nervous system metastases in 10–15% of patients, who have otherwise enjoyed an extended complete or partial remission. A compelling reason to continue radical cystectomy in the adjuvant chemotherapy programmes now under study is the discordance between clinical staging, i.e. T staging including re-TUR-BT, as opposed to P staging, following cystectomy. There is about a 30% error rate between clinical T staging and P staging after cystectomy. This error rate is unacceptable, and bladder sparing on the basis of postchemotherapy clinical staging alone at this point is treacherous.[16,17]

Testis cancer

This type of tumour is remarkable in terms of demonstrating the impact of regional lymphadenectomy on survival. Over the years, many series have shown that node-positive patients can be cured with local measures in excess of 50% of the time. A variety of anatomical considerations, relating to features of the anatomical descent of the gonad and its associated lymphatics, make testicular lymphatic drainage predictable. A number of topographic studies have supported the regional deposition of metastatic disease, and this is now well understood. More importantly, various biological considerations probably improve the opportunity for cure in testis cancer patients with surgery alone. In many patients there will be teratomatous elements, which have a slightly lower metastatic potential. What is fascinating, however, is that even undifferentiated germ cell tumours, such as embryonal cancer, are often cured with lymphadenectomy alone. In a cooperative study, in a control group treated with node dissection alone one-half of the patients were long-term survivors without relapse.[18] Fortunately, the relapsers (with only one exception) were rescued at the time of relapse. The overall survival in stage II disease including all levels of involvement, both stage IIA and IIB is 97.5%. This has been achieved with the use of either adjuvant chemotherapy following retroperitoneal lymph node dissection (RPLND) or observation only for stage II disease.

When considering RPLND procedures the general treatment philosophy should be as follows. The surgery should be appropriate ('let the punishment fit the crime'). Although at present, the author's position in low-stage low-volume disease is divergent from that of those committed to surveillance only, the paths are likely to converge in future. Clearly, no one wants to perform staging RPLND for its own sake. If the clinical sensitivity of clinical staging can attain levels of confidence exceeding the 90th percentile, staging RPLND will become unnecessary. Meanwhile, however, a good interim position is the modified RPLND, particularly that employing nerve-sparing techniques. Virtually all patients who undergo nerve-sparing modified RPLND will be able to ejaculate;[19] thus, the patients has not been harmed, and he has also been adequately staged. In fact, those of the author's patients who do have microscopic disease are also given therapy. At this point, the relapse rate locally in patients with nerve-sparing RPLND is entirely satisfactory in the author's current small and selected series.

Regarding high-stage disease, reviews are generally concordant worldwide. Disseminated disease requires disseminated treatment first. This implies pretreatment with systemic chemotherapy, which is platinum based. Currently, programmes employing platinum (VP-16), with or without bleomycin, are popular and effective. Surgery is reserved for those who have residual clinical disease as noted on the CT scan. One current challenge is to develop predictive criteria for those who might have scar tissue and necrosis only in the specimen.[20,21] There is some analogy with the seminoma data for advanced disease, where it has been found that most patients with a partial remission can be followed because they will have necrosis only in their tissue specimen. However, there are always exceptions to the rule and they must be followed carefully, and any relapse treated aggressively.

Another philosophical point that will affect future management of node dissection in testis cancer is that healthcare providers will want to eliminate qualitative variables in treatment programmes as much as possible. Surgery is always a variable in this regard. In order to simplify and codify quantitative aspects of treatment, there will be a move to eliminate initial hospital costs in such things as staging and/or treatment for low-stage disease. Systemic chemotherapy is more easily standardized and quantified. In some countries, therefore, surgery for low-volume disease will be entirely bypassed and reversed for salvage after chemotherapy. This will require many patients with low-volume disease, limited to the retroperitoneum, to undergo systemic chemotherapy, which has been demonstrated to have negative long-term consequences on their fertility. Primary germ cell damage is well known in patients treated for advanced disease and only about one-half of the author's patients regenerate a satisfactory sperm count after 2–3 years. The systemic approach in clinical low-stage settings will result in treatment excess for many with confined low-volume disease. It would be much simpler to treat low-volume regional disease with regional treatment (i.e. surgery). Current cost–benefit and risk–benefit studies support the role of surgery in clinical stage II disease and even in clinical stage I.[22,23]

In the author's opinion, surgery should be more proactive than reactive in the treatment of low-stage disease. Surgery can cure stage II disease within hours. When it does not do so, a cure is available at that juncture, should the patient relapse; such a relapse is almost always in a pulmonary mode, which is easily detectable and treatable. Again, this is the only solid tumour that is curable by surgery alone more than 50% of the time when the regional nodes are positive. Approach to the retroperitoneum is even more feasible and less harmful in the long term with the development of anatomical nerve-sparing dissections, which preserve ejaculation; this gives an active alternative to surveillance that appears to be quite effective and reasonable. Recent cost–benefit and risk–benefit analyses in clinical stage I and II non-seminomatous germ cell testis cancer support the surgical approach.[22,23]

Finally, concerning high-stage disease, there is general agreement that all tumours persisting after initial chemotherapy should be removed. The author has noted that certain patients with very favourable response criteria can be followed very actively with expectation of further resolution of their radiographic changes.[20,21] The hope is of being more selective in choosing patients for surgery after chemotherapy; if there is any significant concern about the presence of persistent tumour, as a general principle, such patients are more safely managed with exploration and RPLND. Currently, following primary chemotherapy with this approach in over 600 RPLND procedures, 44% of patients have necrosis/fibrosis only, 44% have teratoma, and 12% have cancer. The former two groups are carefully observed postoperatively and the last group with persistent cancer receive two courses of salvage chemotherapy. The overall survival of this group is good (80–90%), but factors predicting for relapse are bulk of tumour, histology, and site (primary mediastinum).[24] Overall, a number of viable options are available in selecting therapy for testis cancer which, if rigorously applied, will yield good results.[25,26]

References

1. deKernion J B. Lymphadenectomy for renal cell carcinoma: therapeutic implications. Urol Clin North Am 1980; 7: 697
2. Peters P C, Brown G L. The role of lymphadenectomy in renal cell carcinoma. Urol Clin North Am 1980; 7: 705
3. Robson C J, Churchill B M, Anderson W. The results of radical nephrectomy for renal cell carcinoma. J Urol 1969; 101: 297
4. Gottesman J E, Crawford E D, Grossman H B. Infarction nephrectomy for metastatic renal cell carcinoma. Urology 1985; 25: 248
5. Fowler J W, Smith M F. Radical nephrectomy; an assessment of morbidity, local control of disease and its effect on prognosis. Br J Urol 1980; 52: 84
6. Guiliani L, Martorana G, Gilberti C et al. Results of radical nephrectomy with extensive lymphadenectomy for renal cell carcinoma. J Urol 1983; 130: 664
7. Pizzocaro G, Piva L, Salvioni R. Lymph node dissection in radical nephrectomy for renal cell carcinoma: is it necessary? Eur Urol 1983; 9: 10
8. Marshall F F, Powell K C. Lymphadenectomy for renal cell carcinoma: anatomical and therapeutic considerations. J Urol 1982; 128: 677
9. Flanigan R C. The failure of infarction and/or nephrectomy in stage IV renal cell cancer to influence survival or metastatic regression. Urol Clin North Am 1987; 14: 757
10. Grabstalt H, Whitmore W F, Melamed M R. Renal pelvic tumors. JAMA 1971; 218: 845
11. Johansson S, Wahlquist L. A prognostic study of urothelial renal pelvic tumors. Cancer 1979; 43: 2525
12. Paulson D F. The prognostic role of lymphadenectomy in adenocarcinoma of the prostate. Urol Clin North Am 1980; 7: 615

13. Grabstalt H. Controversies concerning lymph node dissection for carcinoma of the penis. Urol Clin North Am 1980; 7: 793

14. Mukamel E, deKernion J B. Early versus delayed lymph node dissection in carcinoma of the penis. Urol Clin North Am 1987; 14: 707

15. Johnson D E, Lo R K. Management of regional lymph nodes in penile carcinoma. Five year results following therapeutic groin dissections. Urology 1984; 24: 308–311

16. Skinner D G. Management of invasive bladder cancer: a meticulous pelvic node dissection can make a difference. J Urol 1982; 128: 34

17. Benson M, Olsson C. Bladder cancer. In Paulson D (ed) Genitourinary surgery. Vol. 1. New York: Churchill Livingstone, 1984; 271–312

18. Williams S D, Stablein D M, Einhorn L H *et al.* Immediate adjuvant chemotherapy versus observation with treatment at relapse in pathological stage II testicular cancer. New Engl J Med 1987; 317: 1433

19. Donohue J P, Foster R S, Geier G *et al.* Preservation of ejaculation following nerve-sparing retroperitoneal lymphadenectomy (RPLND). J Urol 1990; 144: 287

20. Donohue J P *et al.* Correlation of CT changes and histological findings in 80 patients having RPLND after chemotherapy for testis cancer. J Urol 1987; 137: 1176

21. Steyerberg E, Keizer J *et al.* Prediction of residual mass histology following chemotherapy for metastatic nonseminomatous germ cell tumour. J Clin Oncol 1995; in press

22. Donohue J P, Thornhill J A, Foster R S *et al.* The role of retroperitoneal lymphadenectomy in clinical stage B testis cancer: the Indiana University experience. J Urol 1995; 153: 85

23. Baniel J, Roth B, Foster R, Donohue J P. Cost and risk benefit in management of clinical stage I and II non-seminomatous germ cell testis cancer. J Surg Oncol 1995; in press

24. Loehrer P J *et al.* Teratoma following chemotherapy for NSGCT testis cancer: a clinicopathological correlation. J Urol 1986; 135: 1183

25. Donohue J P. Options in the management of low stage testicular cancer. AUA Update Ser 1987; Lesson 27, Vol. VI

26. Donohue J P. Selecting initial therapy in seminoma and non-seminoma. Cancer 1987; 60: 490

Kidney

II

Lymph node surgery in renal cell carcinoma: anatomical and therapeutic dilemmas

2

H. G. van der Poel P. F. A. Mulders
F. M. J. Debruyne

Introduction

At the time of diagnosis approximately 50% of patients with renal cell carcinoma present with metastatic disease.[1] Moreover, metastases develop during follow-up in 30–50% of patients presenting with localized disease.[2] Hence, the majority of patients with renal cell cancer encounter metastatic disease during the course of the illness. Since the 3-year survival rate of patients with metastatic disease does not exceed 15%, owing to the lack of effective treatment modalities, therapeutic intervention is aimed at preventing metastases or resecting them at an early (i.e. microscopic) stage. Surgery on the primary tumour remains the first choice of treatment in patients with localized disease. Many studies discuss the additional use of lymphadenectomy to find and resect possible lymph node metastases. Several arguments for this type of treatment are mentioned: (1) tumour staging;[3] (2) reducing the local recurrence rate;[4] (3) prevention of distant metastases.[5] Here, the literature on lymphadenectomy for renal cancer is reviewed.

Anatomy

In 1935, Parker[6] described the anatomy of the lymphoid drainage of the kidney. In right-sided tumours, the first nodes involved are precaval, retrocaval and interaortocaval. For tumours on the left side the first nodes are the para-aortic, preaortic and retroaortic. In a review article, Marshall and Powell[7] recommended a detailed, accurate evaluation of metastases in all patients before surgery, to perform a lymphadenectomy and subsequent pathological investigation of the nodes removed (Table 2.1). Three lymphatic drainage channels exit in the right kidney:

N_0	No identifiable nodes in the specified clinical assessment
N_1	Metastasis in single lymph node, 2 cm or less in greatest dimension
N_2	Metastasis in single lymph node, 2 cm but not more than 5 cm in greatest dimension; in multiple lymph nodes, none more than 5 cm in greatest dimension
N_3	Metastasis in a lymph node more than 5 cm in greatest dimension

Table 2.1. TNM classification for lymph node metastases

anterior, posterior, and middle (Fig. 2.1). For the left kidney, an anterior and posterior drainage channel were described.[7]

(a)   (b)

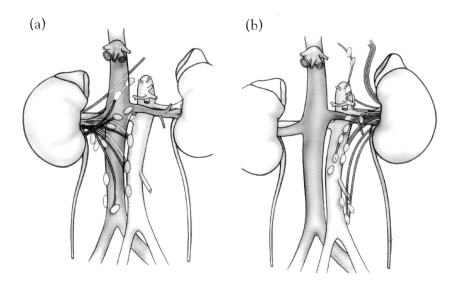

Figure 2.1. Schematic anatomy of lymph channels in (a) right and (b) left kidney. (Reproduced from ref. 12, with permission.)

Lymph node metastases

In localized disease, after radical tumour nephrectomy the 5-year survival rate ranges from 50 to 90% and is dependent on initial tumour stage, tumour size and condition of the patient.[5,8,9] Nurmi[10] found decreased survival in patients with $N+M_0$ disease compared with metastasis-free patients (10 vs 70% 5-year survival). Comparable data were found in a retrospective analysis of 121 patients after radical nephrectomy and lymphadenectomy[9] (Fig. 2.2). In a multivariate analysis, however, lymph

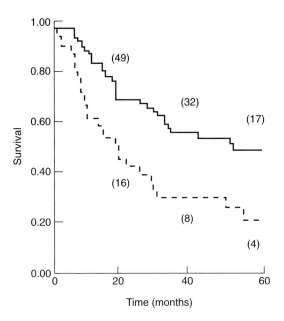

Figure 2.2. Survival after nephrectomy and lymphadenectomy in renal cell carcinoma (n = 121): ——, N_0 (n = 81); – – –, N+ (n = 40). *Difference between N_0 and N+ 5-year survival statistically significant* (p < 0.01; Wilcoxon test).

node metastasis was not an independent prognostic marker over tumour stage.[10] The number of positive lymph nodes in the lymphadenectomy specimen was not correlated with survival.[5]

Lymphadenectomy procedure

In general, extended lymphadenectomy reveals most information on the presence of lymph node metastases.[11] In Figure 2.3 the anatomical boundaries are presented. In particular, on the right side a regional lymph node dissection (removal of the paracaval lymph nodes) is insufficient, since the common sites of metastases are interaortocaval and retrocaval.[12] Extended lymphadenectomy is, therefore, the procedure of choice in several studies.[5,7,8] The resection can be performed at the time of radical nephrectomy and will prolong surgery time by 45–60 min. 'En bloc' resection of the lymph nodes should be aimed for. This can best be done by dissecting close to the larger vessels. In the cranial–caudal plane, dissection should be performed from the diaphragmatic crux down to the bifurcation of the aorta.[12] Lymphatic leakage can be prevented by clipping the lymphatic ducts. As opposed to extended lymphadenectomy, several studies,[8,13] discuss the use of local or even hilar dissection of the

(a)   (b)

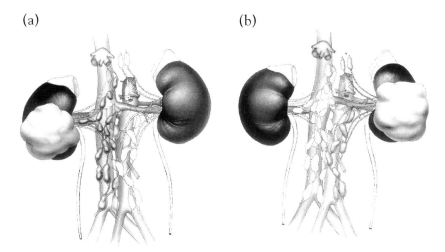

Figure 2.3. Extended lymphadenectomy in (a) right and (b) left kidney. (Reproduced from ref. 12, with permission.)

lymph nodes. The advantages and disadvantages of both techniques are discussed below.

The presence of supradiaphragmatic lymph node metastases is, in the majority of cases (86%), accompanied by distant metastases in, for example, the lung;[14] hence resection of these nodes is not indicated.

Morbidity and mortality of lymphadenectomy

Most studies present complications in 1–3% of lymph node surgery procedures. Major complications are bleeding of lumbar vessels and postoperative lymphocoele. Hospital stay and complication rate do not differ between local and extended lymphadenectomy.[4,15] Mortality rates seem comparable to those found in radical tumour nephrectomy.[5,8,16]

Prognosis and lymphadenectomy

Although the presence of lymph node metastases at the time of tumour nephrectomy indicates a poor prognosis, the role of lymphadenectomy as a therapeutic option is unclear (Table 2.2). The presence of lymph node metastases found after lymphadenectomy ranges from 9 to 32% and seems dependent on the extent of the lymphadenectomy.[8,17–19] The incidence of metastases in extended lymphadenectomy is approximately 25%,[5,20] whereas in regional lymph node resection nodal involvement was found in 15% of cases.[20] Nodal tumour involvement is, in 5–26% of cases, the only sign of metastatic disease.[5,21,22]

Reference	Lymphadenectomy	Stage	5-year survival (%)
Giuliani et al. (1990)[5]	Extended (n=200)	T_1N_0	80
		T_2N_0	68
		T_3N_0	70
		$N+M_0$	52
Herrlinger et al. (1991)[8]	Extended (n=320)	$T_{1-2}N_0$	90
		$T_3N_0V_0$	78
		$N+M_0$	28
	Regional (n=191)	$T_{1-2}N_0$	75
		$T_3N_0V_0$	58
		$N+M_0$	17
Ditonno et al. (1992)[24]	Extended (n=97)	T_1N_0	100
		T_2N_0	79
		T_3N_0	68
		$N+$	25

		Local Recurrence (%)	Progression (%)
Phillips and Messing (1993)[4]	Extended + Regional (n=42)	10	10.5
	N_0(n=27)	3.2	20

*It should be noted that none of the studies was a randomized analysis.

Table 2.2. Survival after nephrectomy with and without lymphadenectomy in recent literature*

The consensus is that lymphadenectomy will be of value only in patients without distant metastases. Peters and Brown[19] found lymphadenectomy of value for survival only in patients with Robson stage C and D disease. Wood[23] hypothesized that extended lymphadenectomy will be of value only in patients with lymph node involvement without distant metastases, i.e. 5–26%. Phillips and Messing,[4] indeed, found reduced local recurrence rates in these patients after lymphadenectomy. However, five of six patients with nodal involvement developed distant metastases despite lymphadenectomy. Similarly, Ditonno et al.[24] did not find improved survival in patients receiving lymphadenectomy for node-positive disease. Herrlinder et al.[8] compared regional or facultative lymph node resection with extended lymphadenectomy in a non-randomized prospective study. In patients receiving extended resection, survival was prolonged compared with regional dissection only for patients with node-negative disease, being highest for patients with $pT_{1-2}N_0M_0$ disease. Interestingly, the survival advantage of extended over regional lymphadenectomy in patients with node-positive disease was present only in the first 3 years after surgery. Overall 10-year survival for both groups was equal.[8] These findings lend support to the theory that lymph node involvement reveals the systemic extent of the disease that can not be cured surgically.[13]

Thus, the survival advantage offered by lymphadenectomy remains to be established. To assess the value of lymphadenectomy a prospective randomized analysis is required. Preoperative lymph node staging, however, will present problems. Although CT scanning offers a reliable method for detecting retroperitoneal adenopathy, lymph node metastases are found in only 31–42% of patients with adenopathy.[4] Moreover, lymph node metastases were found in 6% of cases without pre-or intraoperative adenopathy.[4] In other words, the most reliable method of assessing lymph node status is lymphadenectomy. Preoperative selection of patients eligible for lymphadenectomy will be considered unreliable when lymph node status determined by CT scan is to be taken into account for this selection.

Staging by lymphadenectomy may be the most accurate way to detect nodal tumour involvement, but what is its clinical application? Effective treatment modalities for metastasized renal cell cancer are lacking and new therapies are mainly used in investigative settings. In particular, adjuvant immunotherapy protocols require accurate staging. Hence, lymphadenectomy for staging reasons will be applicable only in an academic setting and is currently of minor clinical implication in day-to-day urology.

Conclusions

On reviewing the literature on lymphadenectomy, the following reasons for this procedure were mentioned: (1) to obtain accurate tumour staging; (2) to reduce the number of local recurrences; (3) to improve overall survival by reducing the risk of distant metastases. Although the local recurrence rate appears to be reduced after lymphadenectomy in node-positive disease, distant metastases occur frequently in these patients. For node-negative disease, extended lymphadenectomy may improve survival by extirpation of microscopic metastases. Lymph node staging by lymphadenectomy is of value only in academic settings, since lymph node status does not implicate therapeutic consequences in patients not included in clinical trials.

In 1992, the European Organization for the Research and Treatment of Cancer (EORTC) terminated a prospective randomized trial (30881) for nephrectomy with or without extended lymphadenectomy. A total of 772 patients, clinically metastasis-free, were randomized. Preliminary data of this study show no difference in side effects between the two groups. Short-term follow-up, however, did not indicate any advantage of extended lymphadenectomy in these patients.[25] The final data from this group of patients will be the first truly randomized study of that kind and will undoubtedly shed light on the use of the procedure. If, at long-term follow-up, the method is judged favourably, its low morbidity rates render it readily applicable in combination with radical nephrectomy.

References

1. Silverberg E, Lubera J. Cancer statistics, 1987. CA 1987; 37: 2
2. Patel N P, Livengood R W. Renal cell cancer: natural history and results of treatment. J Urol 1977; 119: 722
3. Fuselier H A, Guice S L, Brannan W et al. Renal cell carcinoma: the Ochsner Medical Institution experience (1945–1978). J Urol 1983; 130: 445
4. Phillips E, Messing E M. Role of lymphadenectomy in the treatment of renal cell carcinoma. Urology 1993; 41: 9
5. Guiliani L, Giberti C, Martorana G, Rovida S. Radical extensive surgery for renal cell carcinoma: long-term results and prognostic factors. J Urol 1990; 143: 468
6. Parker A E. Studies on the main posterior lymph channels of the abdomen and their connections with lymphatics of the genitourinary system. Am J Anat 1935; 50: 409
7. Marshall F F, Powell K C. Lymphadenectomy for renal cell carcinoma: anatomical and therapeutic considerations. J Urol 1982; 128: 677
8. Herrlinger A, Schrott K M, Schott G, Sigel A. What are the benefits of extended dissection of the regional renal lymph nodes in the therapy of renal cell carcinoma. J Urol 1991; 146: 1224
9. van der Poel H G, Mulders P F A, Oosterhof G O N, et al. Prognostic value of karyometric and clinical characteristics in renal cell carcinoma: quantitative assessment of tumor heterogenity. Cancer 1993; 72: 2667
10. Nurmi M J. Prognostic factors in renal cell carcinoma. An evaluation of operative finding. Br J Urol 1984; 56: 270
11. Saitoh H, Nakayama K, Satoh T. Distant metastasis of renal adenocarcinoma in nephrectomized cases. J Urol 1982; 127: 1092
12. Giuliani L. Lymphadenectomy. In: Atlas of surgery for renal cell cancer. Genoa, 1989: 43–46
13. Simonovitch J P, Monti J E, Straffon R A. Lymphadenectomy in renal adenocarcinoma. J Urol 1982; 127: 1090

14. Hellsten S, Berge T, Linell F, Wehlin L. Clinically unrecognized renal cell carcinoma. An autopsy study. In: Renal tumours. Proc 1st Int Symp on kidney tumors. New York: Alan R. Liss, 1982: 273

15. Carmignani G, Begrano E, Puppo, P et al. Lymphadenectomy in renal cancer. In: Pavone-Mucaluso M, Smith P H (eds) Cancer of the prostate and kidney. NATO Advanced Science Institutes Series. Plenum: New York; 1983: 645

16. Swanson D A, Borges P M. Complications of transabdominal radical nephrectomy for renal cell carcinoma. J Urol 1983; 129: 704

17. Robson C J. Staging of renal cell carcinoma. In: Progress in clinical and biological research. Renal tumors. Proc 1st Int Symp on kidney tumors. New York: Alan R. Liss, 1982; 100: 439

18. Middleton R G, Presto A J. Radical thoracoabdominal nephrectomy for renal cell carcinoma. J Urol 1973; 110: 36

19. Peters P C, Brown G L. The role of lymphadenectomy in the management of renal cell carcinoma. Urol Clin North Am 1980; 7: 705

20. Pizzocaro G, Piva L, Salvioni R. Lymph node dissection in radical nephrectomy for renal cell carcinoma: is it necessary? Eur Urol 1983; 9: 10

21. Skinner D B, Colvin R B, Vermillion C D et al. Diagnosis and management of renal cell carcinoma: a clinical and pathologic study of 309 cases. Cancer 1971; 28: 1165

22. Waters W B, Richie J P. Aggressive surgical approach to renal cell carcinoma: review of 130 cases. J Urol 1979; 122: 306

23. Wood D P. Role of lymphadenectomy in renal cell carcinoma. Urol Clin North Am 1991; 18: 421

24. Ditonno O, Traficante A, Battaglia M et al. Role of lymphadenectomy in renal cell carcinoma. Prog Clin Biol Res 1992; 378: 169

25. Blom J H M, Schröder F H, van Poppel H et al. and the EORTC Genitourinary Group. The therapeutic value of lymph node dissection in conjunction with radical nephrectomy in non-metastastic renal cancer — results of an EORTC phase III study. EAU Proc, 13–16 July. Berlin: ICC, 1994; 313 (abstr 597)

Retroperitoneal lymph node dissection in renal cell carcinoma

3

L. Giuliani[†]   F. Oneto   C. Giberti
G. Martorana   R. Franchini   M Cussotto
S. Rovida   G. Carmignani

Introduction

Renal cell carcinoma has an incidence of about 4.1–5.6 per 100 000 and it mainly affects adults between 50 and 70 years of age, with a male/female ratio of 3:1;[1] it may spread both by direct infiltration and by the bloodstream and/or lymphatic system, and has a marked tendency to extend through the renal vein into the vena cava up to the right atrium.[2]

Approximately one-third of patients already have metastases at diagnosis; the most frequent sites are the lungs, lymph nodes, skeleton, brain and liver.[3]

Nodal metastases are generally considered to be indicators of systemic tumour spread and of poor outcome;[4] however, their precise role in renal cell carcinoma is still unclear, and extensive data are still lacking.[5] This is due to several factors: first, until recent years most of the reported series used the four-stage system as modified by Petkovic[6] and Robson,[7] which groups both regional nodal involvement and renal vein invasion into the same stage III, instead of using the TNM system that provides more analytical information;[8] second, the preoperative diagnosis of lymph node metastases is highly unreliable, since a high percentage of nodal metastases are microscopic in size; third, lymphadenectomy, and especially extended lymphadenectomy, is not accepted as a routine procedure by many surgeons. Moreover, few of the surgeons who perform lymphadenectomy provide information on its extent.

[†]Deceased

Lymphatic drainage of the kidney

The perinephric lymph nodes and regional lymphatics of the kidneys were first described by Mascagni in 1787.[4] Most of the information on regional lymphatic drainage is based on the anatomical works of Poirier,[9] Rouvière[10] and Alice Parker;[11] an excellent, more recent review is by Marshall and Powell.[12]

The results of these anatomical studies can be summarized as follows: the retroperitoneal lymph nodes from the diaphragm down to the aortic bifurcation are the true primary lymph centre of the kidneys; in greater detail, the primary lymph centre of the right kidney is represented by the retro-, para-, pre- and interaortocaval nodes, while the primary lymph centre of the left kidney is represented by the retro-, para- and preaortic nodes.

This, as already described elsewhere, is the extent to which the retroperitoneal lymph nodes are dissected by the authors during transabdominal radical nephrectomy for renal cell carcinoma.[13]

Incidence of retroperitoneal lymph node metastases

The incidence of retroperitoneal lymph node metastases ranges from 4 to 43% (Table 3.1). These extremely variable rates are at least partially due to the extent of lymphadenectomy, as clearly shown by Sigel et al., who reported an incidence of retroperitoneal metastases of 4% in patients undergoing translumbar nephrectomy without lymphadenectomy, of 14% in patients undergoing transperitoneal nephrectomy without formal lymphadenectomy, and of 29% in patients undergoing transperitoneal nephrectomy with formal lymph node dissection.[27] Similarly, Herrlinger et al. found that the incidence of lymph node metastases increased from 10% if a facultative lymph node dissection was performed (only macroscopically suspected nodes removed for staging purposes) to 17.5% if a complete lymph node dissection was undertaken.[28] That the incidence of nodal metastases is directly related to the extent of lymphadenectomy is also supported by the fact that the highest incidence is that reported by Saitoh, who found 45% of nodal involvement in an autopsy study.[26]

A further factor that influences the incidence of nodal metastases relates to the false negative results of routine pathological examination. Fisher et al., reporting on nodal metastases in breast cancer, showed that careful step sectioning of lymph nodes revealed an incidence of occult metastases of up to 24% in patients whose lymph nodes had been judged as negative on routine examination.[30]

More recently, the incidence of nodal metastases has been influenced by the fact that the diagnosis of renal cell carcinoma is often made at an

Author	Reference no.	No. of cases	N+ (%)
Skinner *et al.* (1972)	14	309	6.0
Peters and Brown (1980)	15	356	7.9
Rafia (1970)	16	190	8.0
Siminovitch *et al.* (1982)	17	102	9.0
Middleton and Presto (1973)	18	62	11.0
Tsukamoto *et al.* (1990)	19	102	21.0
Giuliani *et al.* (1994)	–*	328	20.4
Robson *et al.* (1969)	20	88	22.7
Giuliani *et al.* (1992)	21	244	23.8
Waters and Richie (1979)	22	67	24.0
Flocks and Kadesky (1958)	23	137	25.0
Hulten *et al.* (1969)	24	22	32.0
Giuliani *et al.* (1983)	25	106	32.0
Saitoh *et al.* (1982)	26	1828†	45.0
Sigel *et al.* (1981)	27	50‡	4.0
		130§	14.0
		176·	29.0
Herrlinger *et al.* (1991)	28	191¶	10.0
		320**	17.5
Blom *et al.* (EORTC) (1992)	29	313**	5.0

*Present report; †autopsies; ‡translumbar; §transabdominal, no formal lymph node dissection (LND);
·transabdominal with formal LND; ¶faculative LND; **complete LND.

Table 3.1 Incidence of retroperitoneal lymph node metastases in renal cell carcinoma

earlier stage. In the authors' series the incidence has decreased from 32% in 1983 (ref. 25) to 23.8% in 1992 (ref. 21) and 21.3% in 1994 (present report), without any alteration in surgical technique.

In the authors' series there was a significant relationship between the incidence of nodal metastases and the local stage of the tumour, the presence of distant metastases and/or the presence of venous involvement, although the correlation coefficient and Spearman's rho value are not as high (Tables 3.2–3.4). This implies that the clinical stage of the tumour is not a reliable predictor of lymph node involvement in the individual patient and therefore it is not a criterion of the advisability of retroperitoneal lymphadenectomy.

Stage	No. of patients	pN+		pN + M_0V_0	
		(No.)	(%)	(No.)	(%)
pT_1	32	4	12.5	2	6.3
pT_2	135	13	9.6	7	5.2
pT_3	145	45	31.0	14	9.7
pT_4	12	4	33.3	–	–
pT_x	4	1	25.0	–	–
Total	328	67	20.4	23	7.0

Table 3.2. Incidence of nodal metastases in relation to tumour stage

	T	G	N	M	V
T	1	0.279	0.199	0.235	0.348
G	0.279	1	0.205	0.202	0.228
N	0.199	0.205	1	0.294	0.203
M	0.235	0.202	0.294	1	0.174
V	0.348	0.228	0.203	0.174	1

*From 251 valid observations; other cases lost owing to missing data.

Table 3.3. TNMVG correlation matrix*

	Rho	p-value
T	0.475	< 0.0001
G	0.473	< 0.0001
M	0.650	< 0.0001
V	0.577	< 0.0001

Table 3.4. Spearman rank correlation for lymph node involvement (N) with tumour stage (T), tumour grade (G), distant metastases (M) and venous involvement (V)

Characteristics of retroperitoneal lymph node metastases

Retroperitoneal lymph node metastases usually are ipsilateral to the tumour. No patients were found with contralateral positive nodes in the absence of ipsilateral nodal metastases. Contralateral lymph nodes may become involved if multiple ipsilateral metastases are present, which occurs in about 70% of patients with positive nodes.[19]

In the author's series 85% of nodal metastases were microscopic in size; this is similar to the 77% incidence of microscopic nodal involvement reported by Peters and Brown.[15]

Localization of retroperitoneal nodal metastases

The results of the authors' series are shown in Table 3.5; they confirm the finding of Tsukamoto, that the distribution of nodal metastases usually follows the normal lymphatic drainage pathways.[19]

It should be emphasized that the hilar nodes are involved in fewer cases than are the paracaval nodes (for right tumours) or the para-aortic nodes (for left tumours). This clearly indicates that the retroperitoneal lymph nodes are the true primary lymph centre of the kidney whereas the hilar nodes are merely satellite nodes. This is in accordance with the findings of Saitoh et al., who reported that the incidence of metastases in the hilar nodes was only 7% in contrast to 26.8% in the para-aortic nodes and 36% in the paracaval nodes.[26]

Experience of the Urology Clinic of Genoa

From January 1970 to July 1993, 369 consecutive patients underwent radical surgery for renal cell carcinoma (RCC), 41 of which were lost to follow-up; only the remaining 328 patients, therefore, were included in a statistical study.

All but 14 patients with multiple distant metastases underwent wide-field radical nephrectomy with extended lymphadenectomy according to

Right tumours*			Left tumours[†]		
	Patients			Patients	
Nodes involved	No.	%	Nodes involved	No.	%
Hilar	9	27.2	Hilar	12	35.3
Precaval	7	21.2	Preaortic	5	14.7
Retrocaval	9	27.2	Retroaortic	11	32.4
Laterocaval	4	12.1	Lateroaortic	11	32.4
Interaortocaval	15	45.5	Interaortocaval	5	14.7
Others	3	9.1	Others	4	11.8

*33 patients pN+; [†]34 patients pN+.

Table 3.5. Distribution of nodal metastases in the retroperitoneum

the technique described previously.[13,25] Patients ranged in age from 18 to 88 years, with an average of 60 years and a median of 61. There were 217 men and 111 women. The right kidney was involved in 172 patients and the left in 156. TNM was used (IDC-O-189.0, First Edition, 1978); the pathological staging of the tumours is reported in Table 3.6.

Prognostic significance of lymph node metastases: role and extent of retroperitoneal lymphadenectomy

Patient survival was calculated by the life table Kaplan–Meier method and differences in survival were evaluated by means of the log rank test. The cumulative overall survival rate after radical nephrectomy and extended lymphadenectomy in this series was 50.7, 35.1 and 29% at 5, 10 and 15 years, respectively.

In patients with tumour stage $pT_1N_0M_0V_0$, the survival rate at 5, 10 and 15 years was 90, 64.2 and 53.5%, respectively, while in patients with tumour stage $pT_2N_0M_0V_0$ the rate was 74.9, 52.8 and 43.2%, again at 5, 10 and 15 years, respectively.

There was a 6.6% incidence of nodal metastases in patients with tumour apparently confined to the kidney $(T_1–T_2M_0V_0)$. Consequently, it is evident that in low-stage tumours also, radical nephrectomy plus extended lymphadenectomy may have a potentially curative role and is essential for staging the tumour correctly. Furthermore, if careful step sectioning of the lymph nodes is performed, it is likely that, according to Fisher et al.,[30] a significant percentage of the patients that are diagnosed as pN_0 at routine pathological examination would be upstaged to pN+, particularly in low T-stage tumours. In the authors' opinion, therefore,

pT_1	= 32	$pT_1N_0M_0V_0$	= 28
pT_2	= 135	$pT_2N_0M_0V_0$	= 102
pT_3	= 145	$pT_3N_0M_0V_0$	= 47
pT_4	= 12	$pT_4N_0M_0V_0$	= 0
pT_X	= 4		
pN_0	= 247		
pN+	= 67	$pN+M_0V_0$	= 23
pN_X	= 14		
M_1	= 77		
M_X	= 4		
V+	= 79	$V+N_0M_0$	= 35

Table 3.6. TNM classification of 328 evaluable patients from a total of 369 patients undergoing surgery for renal cell adenocarcinoma (1970–1993)

not performing an extended lymphadenectomy also in patients with low T-stage tumour would expose them to a significant risk of local recurrence or of appearance of distant metastases arising from the microscopic lymph node metastases that are left in situ.

Patients with tumour extending to perirenal fat $(T_3N_0M_0)$ have shown 75.8 and 41.2% survival rates at 5 and 10 years. These figures are even better than the 47% 5-year survival rate reported by Skinner and represent a significant improvement over the 14% registered with simple nephrectomy.[31]

In patients with lymph node metastases $(N_{1-3}M_0V_0)$ the survival rate was 47.9 and 31.9% at 5 and 10 years, respectively. This survival rate is significantly higher than that of patients with distant metastases $(p < 0.05)$ and, from the clinical and practical standpoint, is not very different from that of patients with involvement of the perirenal fat $(T_3N_0M_0)$, although a statistically significant difference has been demonstrated in this last review of the series (0.05; log rank test).

A higher 5-year survival rate was found in patients with fewer than two nodes involved (51.6%) than in those with more than two nodes involved (21.4%), although this difference does not reach statistical significance owing to the limited number of patients. In future it would be of interest to stratify patients according to the size of nodal metastases. In fact, the present results may have been influenced by the fact that 85% of nodal metastases in the series were microscopic.

The actuarial survival in this series is clearly superior to those reported by authors who do not perform extended lymphadenectomy, and who obtain 5-year survival rates in patients with positive nodes ranging from 11 to 21%.[8,16,17,32] Robson, who does perform extended lymphadenectomy, reports 5- and 10-year survival rates of 35%.[20]

The importance of the extent of lymphadenectomy is confirmed by the comparative study by Peters and Brown,[15] who found that patients with stage C renal cancer had a survival rate of 44 or 26%, respectively, depending on whether they did or did not undergo retroperitoneal lymphadenectomy. Golimbu and associates reported a difference in 5-year survival rates between patients with stage II disease who underwent lymphadenectomy and those who did not (80 vs 65%, respectively). In addition, patients with stage III renal cancer and renal vein involvement alone subjected to lymph node dissection had a better survival rate than those not subjected to lymphadenectomy (60% vs 47%, respectively). The authors concluded that the improvement in survival associated with lymphadenectomy is probably due to the removal of micrometastases.[3]

Herrlinger et al., in a prospective study, evaluated 511 patients who underwent radical nephrectomy for RCC. Of these, 320 underwent complete lymph-node dissection, whereas in the other 191 patients only a facultative lymphadenectomy was performed which means that only macroscopically suspected nodes were removed for staging. These authors reported a statistically significant difference in survival ($p < 0.01$) among patients with stage I and II RCC depending on whether lymphadenectomy had been complete (stage I, 80.2% 10-year survival; stage II, 58.2% 10-year survival) or incomplete (stage I, 54% 10-year survival; stage II, 41.2% 10-year survival).[28] No advantage of extended lymphadenectomy was observed for Robson stage III disease, and these authors concluded that macroscopic invasion of the tumour into the renal veins had overcome the assumed curative effect of extended lymph node dissection.[28]

Conversely, other authors consider complete lymph node dissection to be of no therapeutic value in the treatment of RCC. Thus, Pizzocaro et al. stated that lymph node involvement is expected to be present in about 16–18% of patients with operable M_0 RCC and that surgical cure of N+ patients does not exceed 35% even in the most favourable circumstances. Hence, at most, 6% of these patients will benefit from lymphadenectomy.[33] Bassil et al. performed a retrospective analysis of 252 patients with RCC and compared the survival rate of 100 patients who underwent radical nephrectomy with that of 133 patients who underwent radical nephrectomy with extensive regional or para-aortic lymph node dissection. The 5-year survival rate for those patients who underwent radical nephrectomy alone was 59%, compared with 65% for those who had radical nephrectomy and lymphadenectomy. The differences were not statistically significant in either the stage T_2 or the stage T_3 categories.[8] Similarly, Siminovich et al. stated that complete lymph node dissection has no therapeutic value in the treatment of RCC.[17]

The preliminary results of a prospective, randomized, multicentre European Organization for the Research and Treatment of Cancer (EORTC) study, in which 637 patients were entered in 1992, suggest that there are no statistically significant differences in the progression rate of the disease between patients undergoing complete lymphadenectomy (6.7%) and those receiving only radical nephrectomy without lymphadenectomy (5.2%).[29]

deKernion pointed out that many patients with negative nodes may die of disseminated tumour, indicating that bloodborne metastases are perhaps more frequent causes of death in RCC than are lymphatic metastases. Thus, lymphadenectomy can be justified only if lymphatic metastases are the only extent of tumour dissemination.[34]

Nevertheless, the present authors found an extremely low rate of local tumour recurrence (5/328 patients; 1.5%); it is likely that this was due to the complete removal of regional disease by means of extended lymphadenectomy. Although this is not sufficient to improve survival, it certainly improves the patients' quality of life.

In conclusion, these results further confirm the authors' previous findings,[25,35] that lymphadectomy, and extended lymphadenectomy in particular, has an important role in the prognosis of patients with nodal metastases only (M_0V_0), since it may be curative in cases of microscopic node involvement, especially in low T-stage tumours. Therefore, as extended lymphadenectomy does not increase operative morbidity and mortality,[28,35,29,36] facilitates improved surgical staging and lowers local tumour recurrence rates, in the authors' opinion it is an integral part of radical nephrectomy.

References

1. Kantor A F. Current concepts in the epidemiology of primary renal cell carcinoma. J Urol 1977; 117: 415
2. Hermanek P, Sigel A, Chlepas S. Renal cell carcinoma: invasion of veins. Eur Urol 1976; 2: 142
3. Golimbu M, Joshi P, Sperberg A et al. Renal cell carcinoma: survival and prognostic factors. Urology 1986; 27: 291
4. Haagensen C D, Feind C R, Grinnel R S et al. The lymphatics in cancer. Philadelphia: Saunders, 1972
5. Giuliani L. Lymphadenectomy and renal cell carcinoma: why is there so much controversy? Eur Urol 1983; 9: 374
6. Petkovic S D. An anatomical classification of renal tumours in the adult as a basis for prognosis. J Urol 1969; 81: 618
7. Robson C J, Churchill B M, Anderson W. The results of radical nephrectomy for renal cell carcinoma. J Urol 1969; 101: 297
8. Bassil B, Dosoretz D E, Prout G R, Jr. Validation of the tumour nodes and metastasis classification of renal cell carcinoma. J Urol 1985; 134: 450
9. Poirier P, Cuneo B, Delamere G. The lymphatics. London: Archibald Constable, 1903
10. Rouvière H. Anatomie des lymphatiques de l'homme. Paris: Masson, 1932
11. Parker A E. Studies on the main posterior lymph-channels of the abdomen and their connections with the lymphatic of the genito-urinary system. Am J Anat 1935; 56: 409
12. Marshall F F, Powell K C. Lymphadenectomy for renal cell carcinoma: anatomical and therapeutic considerations. J Urol 1981; 126: 17
13. Giuliani L. Atlas of surgery for renal cancer, 2nd ed. Milan: Grafiche Mazzucchelli, 1992
14. Skinner D G, Colvin R B, Vermillion C D et al. Diagnosis and management of renal cell carcinoma: a clinical and pathologic study of 309 cases. Cancer 1971; 28: 1165
15. Peters P C, Brown G L. The role of lymphadenectomy in the management of renal cell carcinoma. Urol Clin North Am 1980; 7: 705
16. Rafla S. Renal cell carcinoma: natural history and results of treatment. Cancer 1970; 25: 26

17. Siminovitch J P, Montie J E, Straffon R A. Lymphadenectomy in renal adenocarcinoma. J Urol 1982; 127: 1090
18. Middleton R G, Presto A J. Radical thoracoabdominal nephrectomy for renal cell carcinoma. J Urol 1973; 110: 36
19. Tsukamoto T, Kumamoto Y, Miyao N et al. Regional lymph node metastasis in renal cell carcinoma: incidence, distribution and its relation to other pathologic findings. Eur Urol 1990; 18: 88
20. Robson C J, Churchill B M, Anderson W. The results of radical nephrectomy for renal cell carcinoma. J Urol 1969; 101: 297
21. Giuliani L, Giberti C, Oneto F. Lymph node metastases in renal cell carcinoma. In: EORTC Genitourinary Group Monograph 11: Recent progress in bladder and kidney cancer. New York: Wiley-Liss, 1992: 153–160
22. Waters W B, Richie J P. Aggressive surgical approach to renal cell carcinoma: review of 130 cases. J Urol 1979; 122: 306
23. Flocks R H, Kadesky M C. Malignant neoplasm of the kidney: an analysis of 350 patients followed five years or more. J Urol 1958; 79: 196
24. Hulten L, Rosencrantz M, Seeman T et al. Occurence and localization of lymph node metastases in renal cell carcinoma. A lymphographic and histopathological investigation in connection with nephrectomy. Scand J Urol Nephrol 1969; 3: 129
25. Giuliani L, Martorana G, Giberti C et al. Results of radical nephrectomy with extensive lymphadenectomy for renal cell carcinoma. J Urol 1983; 130: 664
26. Saitoh H, Nakayama M, Nakamura K, Satoh T. Distant metastasis of renal adenocarcinoma in nephrectomized cases. J Urol 1982; 127: 1092
27. Sigel A, Chlepas S, Schrott K M, Hermanek P. Die operation des nierentumors. Chirurg 1981; 52: 545
28. Herrlinger A, Schrott K M, Schrott G et al. What are the benefits of extended dissection of the regional renal lymph nodes in the therapy of renal cell carcinoma? J Urol 1991; 146: 1224
29. Blom J H M, Schroder F H, Sylvester R, Hammond B. The EORTC Genitourinary Group: The therapeutic value of lymphadenectomy in conjunction with radical nephrectomy in non metastatic renal cancer — results of an EORTC phase III study. J Urol 1992; 147: 422A (abstr)
30. Fisher E R, Swamidoss S, Lee C H. Detection and significance of occult axillary metastases in patients with invasive breast cancer. Cancer 1978; 42: 2025
31. Skinner D G, Vermillion C D, Colvin R B. The surgical management of renal cell carcinoma. J Urol 1972; 107: 705
32. Pizzocaro G, Lymphadenectomy in renal adenocarcinoma. In deKernion J B, Pavone Macaluso M, (eds) Tumors of the kidney: International Perspectives in Urology, Vol. 13. Baltimore: Williams and Wilkins, 1986: 75
33. Pizzocaro G, Piva L. Pros and cons of retroperitoneal lymphadenectomy in operable renal cell carcinoma. Eur Urol 1990; 18(suppl 2): 22
34. deKernion J B. Lymphadenectomy for renal cell carcinoma: therapeutic implications. Urol Clin North Am 1980; 7: 697
35. Giuliani L, Giberti C, Martorana G, Rovida S. Radical extensive surgery for renal cell carcinoma: long term results and prognostic factors. J Urol 1990; 143: 468
36. Wood D P Jr Role of lymphadenectomy in renal cell carcinoma. Urol Clin North Am 1991; 18: 421

Lymphatogenous spread of renal cell carcinoma: an autopsy study

4

J. A. Johnsen   S. Hellsten

Introduction

The natural course of renal cell carcinoma is highly unpredictable. In approximately one-third of all patients with newly diagnosed renal cancer, metastatic spread is found already at presentation. Renal cell carcinoma may spread by local infiltration, via the bloodstream and/or the lymphatic system. The commonest metastatic sites are the lungs, lymph nodes, bones and liver. The incidence of lymph node metastases as reported in the literature ranges from 6%[1] to 45%[2] in an autopsy study. This extreme variation in incidence probably reflects only the extent of lymph node dissection, implying that the true incidence of lymph node metastases in renal cell carcinoma remains unknown.

The uncertainties concerning incidence, extent and clinical significance of lymphatogenous dissemination in renal cell carcinoma indicate a need for further investigation of the natural history and spread of the disease. The aim of the present study was to analyse the occurrence of metastatic spread in patients with clinically unrecognized renal cell carcinoma, particularly in relation to T stage of the primary tumour, and also the metastatic pattern and histopathological findings.

Patients and methods

Between 1958 and 1982, 1063 new cases of renal cell carcinoma were diagnosed in the town of Malmö, Sweden. In 509 patients (48%) the cancer was clinically diagnosed, while the remaining 554 cases were found among a total of 47 352 autopsies performed during the same period. Consequently, these 554 cases of renal cell carcinoma were undetected until the postmortem examination.

Tumour size was used to differentiate between renal cell carcinoma and cortical adenoma, so that tumours measuring 2 cm or more were included in the study. Smaller tumours were included only if they showed signs of aggressive growth, i.e. local infiltration of the tumour, vascular growth and/or metastases, or when the cellular picture agreed with that of a renal cell carcinoma. Vascular tumour growth was defined as infiltration into branches of the renal vein as well as microscopically demonstrated growth into capillary vessels within or in the surroundings of the tumour. Pericapsular growth denoted infiltration into or through the tumour capsule, when present, or into the renal pelvis, the fibrous capsule of the kidney or the perirenal fatty tissue. Presence of lymph node metastases was confirmed by histological examination of paracaval, para-aortic and mediastinal lymph nodes. In most cases the histological examination also included the supraclavicular, axillary and inguinal lymph nodes. Histological examination of all macroscopically suspected extralymphatic metastases was also performed.

Results

Among the 554 patients with clinically unrecognized renal cell carcinoma, metastatic spread to regional and/or distant lymph nodes was demonstrated in 80 cases. Lymphatic spread restricted to the para-aortic and/or paracaval nodes was found in 21 patients, but additional non-lymphatic metastases were found in 16 of these patients; consequently, only five patients were found to have regional lymphatic spread without concomitant distant metastases. Spread to other lymph node stations was always associated with non-lymphatic metastases.

Mediastinal nodes were involved in 52 (65%) of the 80 patients with lymphatic spread, associated with pulmonary metastases in 49 cases (94.2%).

Metastases to supraclavicular, axillary and inguinal nodes were associated with additional lymphatic spread in all but two cases, one with supraclavicular and one with axillary involvement. Both of these two patients, however, had multiple non-lymphatic metastases.

Conclusions

In previous autopsy study from Malmö, Sweden,[3] including 235 cases of clinically unrecognized renal cell carcinoma, the overall incidence of metastatic spread was 24% with involvement of lymph nodes in 16% of cases. In the present investigation, which was an extension of that study, comprising 554 cases of clinically unrecognized renal cell carcinoma diagnosed during a 25-year period, metastases were revealed in 21.5% and lymph node metastases in 14%. These figures for metastatic spread accord well with those of another series of cases of clinically diagnosed renal cell carcinoma.[4]

The present study demonstrated that most metastatic spread was multifocal, a point to be borne in mind when considering surgery in a patient with known metastases. In the authors' opinion, an aggressive surgical approach aiming to remove all neoplastic growth will be beneficial in only a small proportion of patients exhibiting metastases.

The advisability of retroperitoneal lymph node dissection has been discussed for at least 20 years and is still controversial. The reported 5-year survival of 35% after radical nephrectomy with extensive lymph node dissection for metastases[5] may indicate a selection of referred patients, as it has not been possible to reproduce this excellent rate.

In the present series, localized tumour growth was confined to paracaval and/or para-aortic lymph nodes in only five of the 554 patients with clinically unrecognized renal cell carcinoma (0.9%). In the remaining 62 cases with tumour spread to the regional nodes, additional metastases were revealed.

Nodal metastases were restricted to the mediastinum in eight patients, the supraclavicular fossae in one and the axillary region in one patient. In all eight cases with metastases to the mediastinum without growth in the regional nodes, pulmonary metastases were present, and both the patients with more distant lymph node metastases exclusively had massive haematogenous spread of the renal tumour. Such rare single metastases in peripheral lymph nodes should, therefore, be regarded as an expression of bloodborne tumour spread.

On the basis of the present autopsy series, it is concluded that once renal cell carcinoma has spread to the lymphatic system the risk of multifocal spread is extremely high and only a very few patients would benefit from an extensive lymphadenectomy. Consequently, the main indication for a limited, unilateral lymph node dissection, including removal of the retroperitoneal nodes between the level of the adrenal vessels and the origin of the inferior mesenteric artery, as previously described by deKernion,[6] may be considered as a staging procedure. For a few patients with small metastases restricted to the regional lymph nodes, this procedure may also have a curative effect.

References

1. Skinner D G, Colvin R B, Vermillion C D et al. Diagnosis and management of renal cell carcinoma. A clinical and pathologic study of 309 cases. Cancer 1971; 28: 1165–1177
2. Saitoh H, Nakayama M, Nakamura K, Satoh T. Distant metastasis of renal adenocarcinoma in nephrectomized cases. J Urol 1982; 127: 1092
3. Hellsten S, Berge T, Linell F. Clinically unrecognized renal cell carcinoma: aspects of tumour morphology, lymphatic and haematogenous metastatic spread. Br J Urol 1983; 55: 166–170

4. Ritchie AWS. Current treatment approaches to renal cell carcinoma — the role of surgery. In: Kaye S B (ed) Progress in the treatment of renal cell carcinoma. Proceedings, National Symposium, Cambridge, 31 March 1989. Egham: Medical Action Communications

5. Robson C J, Churchill B M, Anderson W. The results of radical nephrectomy for renal cell carcinoma. J Urol 1969; 101: 297–301

6. deKernion J B. Lymphadenectomy for renal cell carcinoma. Therapeutic implications. Urol Clin North Am 1980; 7: 697–703

Bladder

Lymph nodes in bladder cancer

5

M. Blas Marin   C. Rioja Sanz
L. A. Rioja Sanz

Introduction

Approximately one-third of patients with bladder cancer present with an infiltrating tumour at diagnosis. Patients with infiltrating tumours continue to be a difficult group to treat despite aggressive treatment including exeresis and adjuvant therapy; approximately 50% die as a result of the tumour within 18 months of surgery.

The iliopelvic lymphatic system is an important route of metastasis for bladder tumours; for this reason, identification of N+ at this level affects not only treatment but also prognosis of the disease. Drainage of the bladder lymphatic system begins at the perivesical fat, continuing to the obturator or hypogastric groups, on to the external iliacs and presacrals, and as far as the primitive iliac and retroperitoneal groups.

The negative effect of node involvement on the survival of patients with infiltrating bladder cancer has been well known for about 50 years, since the publications of Jewett.[1] In 1953, Whitmore indicated that only 21% of patients with N(+) survived the first year and 9% the second.[2,3] Kerr, in 1950, found a lower recurrence rate when cystectomy is associated with lymphadenectomy.[4]

All of the series reviewed are in agreement that univariate or multivariate analyses of the prognostic factors that negatively affect the evolution of infiltrating bladder cancer, pathology staging and node involvement are the most important; pathology grade, L+, aneuploidy, etc. all remain secondary as they do not improve the predictive values.

What is the frequency of node involvement with relation to pathology staging?

In the lower pathology stages and superficial tumours, the incidence of N+ is practically nil (less than 5%), whereas in invasive tumour of the muscles the incidence is between 15 and 30%, and is well over 40% in tumours invading the serosa (Table 5.1). This authors' own series of 204 cystectomies is in accord with the rest of the series, where there is a low

Series	Ref. no.*	No. of patients	pN(+) (%)	Percentage involvement at pathological stage					
				P_{is}/P_a	P_1	P_2	P_{3a}	P_{3b}	P_4
Giuliani	5	93	27		0	9	34		60
Laplante	6	302	18						
Skinner	7	591	22	0.7	13	20	24	42	45
Solsona	8	121	24			9	50		55
Smith	9	662	20	2	1	8	47		42
Wishnow	10	130	14			0	13		27
Rioja†		204	19		6	11	16	39	34

*As in reference list.
†Series reported here.

Table 5.1. Node involvement (pN+) in relation to pathological stage of tumour in patients with bladder cancer.

percentage of involvement for pT_1 and pT_2 (12 and 11%), while reaching 38 and 34% for pT_{3b} and pT_4, respectively.

How far does node involvement affect survival rates? Does the number of nodes affect survival? Are there differences in local tumour recurrence depending on node involvement?

It is known that the presence of N+ indicates an inevitable progression towards death. Equally, this prognosis seems to be clearly related to the extent of node involvement, i.e. the number and volume of nodes involved. Those patients with involvement who survive are found to have only one or two nodes involved, or only microscopic nodes.

Analysis of the authors' series of 204 cystectomies with a global incidence of 80.3% N– versus 19.6% N+, the survival rate at 3 years for N– is 72%, but is only 26% for N+. It is interesting to analyse whether the number of nodes infiltrated significantly affects survival. Performing a Kaplan–Meier actuarial study of survival, significant differences could be found for survival in N_1 compared with N_2 or N_3: whereas 31% survive at 3 years with N_1, only 18% do so with N_2 or N_3, with a statistical significance of $p < 0.05$. However, the survival rate at 5 years is very similar for both groups — 21 and 17%, respectively. Similar findings are reported by various authors who have analysed survival rates at 3 and 5 years. Roehrborn found significant differences in survival between N_1 and N_2 during the first 3 years but no significance at 5 years.[11] Skinner and colleagues obtained a survival rate of 35% at 5 years with involvement of one to five nodes, the survival rate decreasing to 17% with an involvement of six nodes.[7] Grossman has reported a survival of 40% beyond 40 months with N_1 as opposed to a survival rate of 9% when more than one node is involved.[12] Solsona and colleagues[13] found significant differences in actuarial survival of N_1 as opposed to N_2, and between these when compared with N_3 or N_4 (Table 5.2).

Skinner[7] has reported the most important series of N+ patients who underwent radical surgery with a follow-up of more than 10 years: the possibility of survival at 2, 3, 5 and 10 years was 55, 38, 29 and 20%, respectively. He and other authors[9,14,15] obtained a survival rate of approximately 53% at 5 years in those patients with one or two nodes involved; the patients benefiting most from lymphadenectomy were those who had microscopic invasion of a few nodes, with a cure rate of 35%.

With regard to local control of the disease, lymphadenectomy appears to bring about a decrease of local recurrence, the patient dying of metastatic disease with no recurrence at the same location. Kerr and Colby[4] ratify these facts, and Skinner[16] refers in his series to the good local control of the disease as recurrence of cancer is local in only 15/89 patients (17%).

Series	Ref. no.*	No. of Patients	No. of positive nodes	Survival (%)	
				2–3 years	5 years
Roehrborn	11	20	1	30	23.3
		22	>1	18.5	18.5
Skinner	7	132	1–5	61	35
Grossman	12	10	1		40
		11	>1		9
Solsona	13	55	1		45
			>1		7

*As in reference list.

Table 5.2. Effect of node involvement on survival of patients with bladder cancer

Is isolated lymphadenectomy indicated for staging or control of bladder cancer? Will the indications for cystectomy alter the fact of finding not clinically suspected N+?

From the authors' viewpoint, as their group assiduously performs laparoscopic lymphadenectomy for staging in prostate cancer, it is their opinion that the procedure is seldom indicated in this condition. A valid alternative does not exist for palliative conservative treatment of bladder cancer. Even if it is not curative, cystectomy with lymphadenectomy continues to be the best therapeutic option, leading to the best survival rates and local control of the disease. In many of these patients the bladder cancer would not be controlled by conservative endoscopic methods. On the other hand, improvement in the rates of local control of the disease enables these patients to be offered bladder substitution or continent diversion, which is much less irksome than the classic diversions.

In the authors' opinion, lymphadenectomy is currently indicated in two very specific circumstances:

1. To assess the pathological response of patients undergoing neoadjuvant chemotherapy, in order to differentiate between those with a complete response and those with only a partial response and to be able to convert the latter to complete responses by means of surgery. Similarly, it is indicated in those patients included in protocols for the conservation of the bladder, so that the pathological response can be assessed accurately, as conventional methods of node staging have a very high rate of failure.
2. A second situation where cystectomy could be avoided in very exceptional cases where it does not improve either survival rate or local control, is in patients with very undifferentiated neoplasms with high grade and stage of pathology, that are controlled endoscopically, and that are going to cause the death of the patient through generalized metastasis before creating local problems.

Conclusions

We may summarize these observations as follows:

1. Node involvement in infiltrating bladder cancer carries a very poor prognosis;

2. Lymphadenectomy is the most accurate method of staging: it defines the high-risk patient, does not show significant morbidity nor prolong the cystectomy, and allows for surgical exeresis of the tumour;

3. Although the therapeutic aspects of lymphadenectomy have not been touched on here, it should be emphasized that the survival rate for surgery can be improved by 1–10%; the patients most benefiting are those in whom infiltration was not suspected and was microscopic, and in whom few nodes are involved.

4. Lymphadenectomy identifies those patients who could benefit from early adjuvant chemotherapy;

5. Lymphadenectomy provides improved local control of the disease;

6. By analysis of the results obtained in patients undergoing neoadjuvant therapy (radiotherapy or chemotherapy), lymphadenectomy identifies tumours resistant to such therapy.

References

1. Jewett H J, Strong G H. Infiltrating carcinoma of the bladder: relation of depth of penetration of the bladder wall to incidence of local extension and metastases. J Urol 1946; 55: 366

2. Whitmore W F Jr, Marshall V F. Carcinoma of the bladder. Surg Clin North Am 1953; 33: 501

3. Whitmore W F. Le traitement des cancers invasifs de la vessie. J Urol (Paris) 1988; 94: 337

4. Kerr W S Jr, Colby F. H. Pelvic lymphadenectomy and total cystectomy in the treatment of carcinoma of the bladder. J Urol 1950; 63: 842

5. Giuliani L, Giberti C, Martorana et al. Lymphadenectomy during radical cystectomy for bladder cancer. In: Management of advanced cancer of prostate and bladder. Ed Alan R. Liss. 1988: 329

6. Laplante M, Brice N. The upper limits of hopeful application of radical cystectomy for vesical carcinoma: does nodal metastasis always indicate incurability. J Urol 1973; 109: 261

7. Lerner S P, Skinner D G, Lieskovsky G et al. The rationale for en bloc pelvic lymph node dissection for bladder cancer patients with nodal metastases: long-term results. J Urol 1993; 149: 758–765

8. Solsona Narbon E, Monros Lliso J L, Ricos Torrent J V et al. Valor de la afectación de las cadenas linfáticas en el pronóstico y tratamiento de los tumores vesicales infiltrativos. Actas Urol Esp 1987; 11: 192

9. Smith J A, Whitmore W F. Regional lymph node metastases from bladder cancer. J Urol 1981; 126: 591

10. Wishnow K I, Johnson D E, Ro J Y et al. Incidence, extent and location of unsuspected pelvic lymph node metastasis in patients undergoing radical cystectomy for bladder cancer. J Urol 1987; 137: 408

11. Roehrborn C G, Sagalowsky A I and Peters P C. Long-term patient survival after cystectomy for regional metastatic transitional cell carcinoma of the bladder. J Urol 1991; 146: 36

12. Grossman H B, Konnak J W. Is radical cystectomy indicated in patients with regional lymphatic metastases? Urology 1988; 31: 214

13. Ricos J V, Iborra F, Casanova J *et al.* La embolización tumoral de las estructuras vasculo-linfáticas de la pared vesical (L+). Su influencia en la evolución de los tumores vesicales. Arch Esp Urol 1991; 44: 965–969

14. Zincke H, Patterson D E, Utz D C *et al.* Pelvic lymphadenectomy and radical cystectomy for transitional cell carcinoma of the bladder with pelvic nodal disease. Br J Urol 1885; 57: 156

15. Dretler S P, Ragsdale B D, Leadbetter W F. The value of pelvic lymphadenectomy in the surgical treatment of bladder cancer. J Urol 1973; 109: 414

16. Skinner D G. The value of regional lymph node dissection in genitourinary cancer. Semin Surg Oncol 1989; 5: 235

What is the role of pelvic lymph node dissection in bladder cancer?

6

A. Tajima   S. Kameyama
K. Kawabe   Y. Aso   A. Ishikawa
T. Ushiyama   Y. Ohtawara
K. Suzuki   K. Fujita

Introduction

Urologists usually perform pelvic lymph node dissection in conjunction with total cystectomy, without fully considering the reasons for this procedure. What is the role and significance of pelvic lymph node dissection in cases of bladder cancer? To the authors' knowledge, few papers that systematically discuss this question have been published, although new treatments and procedures for bladder cancer, such as neoadjuvant and adjuvant chemotherapies, and laparoscopic pelvic lymphadenectomy are being developed.

In this chapter, the current role and significance of pelvic lymph node dissection in bladder cancer are discussed from the risk–benefit and cost–benefit viewpoints, based on the authors' experience and literature review.

Lymph node metastasis and prognosis

Table 6.1 gives the clinical results of the authors' 255 cases of bladder cancer.[1] The survival rate after the various treatments decreased as the pathological stage of the disease became more advanced. Although the number of cases examined was too small to allow any definitive conclusion to be made, it seems that the prognosis was particularly poor for patients with lymph node metastasis: their 5-year survival rate was only 12%.

Radical cystectomy (which means total cystectomy plus bilateral pelvic lymph node dissection) was performed on 61 cases out of 255. Figure 6.1 shows the relationship between pathological stage and pelvic

43

Stage	No. of patients	Survival rate (%) 3-year	5-year
T_{is}	7	100	67
T_a	43	86	81
T_1	111	86	81
T_2	33	46	35
T_3	19	49	41
T_4	5	46	40
N+	14	12	12

Table 6.1. Clinical results in 255 cases of bladder tumour

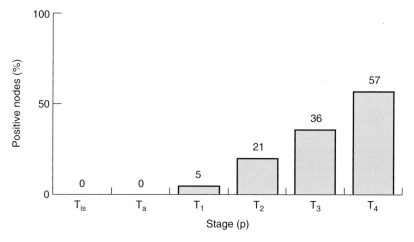

Figure 6.1. Relationship between pathological stage and pelvic lymph node metastasis in 61 patients undergoing total cystectomy plus bilateral pelvic lymph node dissection.

lymph node metastasis for all 61 cases. The percentage of patients with lymph node metastasis increased as the pathological stage became higher: it was 5% for T_1 cases, 21% for T_2, and 36% for T_3; the percentage was as high as 57% for T_4 cases. Figure 6.2 depicts the relationship between tumour grade and pelvic lymph node metastasis for the same population: lymph node metastasis was seen in 27% of G_2 cases and 29% of G_3 cases. Thus, about 30% of patients with high-grade bladder tumour had lymph node metastases.

In reviewing published work concerning the relationship between the prognosis of bladder cancer patients and the presence or absence of pathological lymph node metastases, it is important to distinguish

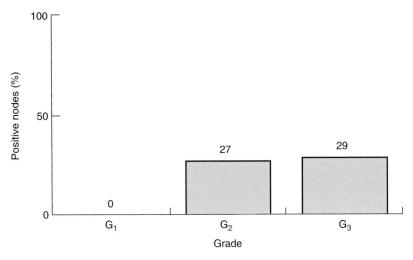

Figure 6.2. Relationship between tumour grade and pelvic lymph node metastasis in the same population as in Figure 6.1.

between clinical lymph node metastases (enlarged metastatic nodes detected by CT scan in a patient with muscle-infiltrating disease) and pathological lymph node metastases (metastases detected only by histopathological examination of the tissues provided by pelvic lymph node dissection). For patients with positive clinical lymph node metastases, it seems appropriate to begin treatment using systemic chemotherapy. It has been reported that lymph node metastases respond better to chemotherapy than do metastases of other organs.[2]

Most previous reports dealing with the relationship between prognosis and pathological lymph node metastasis indicate that the prognosis is poorer in patients with pathological lymph node metastasis, and that the incidence of lymph node metastasis increases as the stage of the disease becomes higher.[3–5] They also indicate that the prognosis is poorer as the number of metastatic lesions increases. These findings are fundamentally consistent with the findings obtained in the present authors' series. On the basis of these findings, the role of pelvic lymph node dissection may be said to be to enable surgeons to estimate the prognosis of the patient with bladder cancer through histopathological examination of the lymph node removed. The results indicate the prognosis: patients with positive nodes have a dismal prognosis.

Extent and therapeutic effect of lymph node dissection

What should be the extent of lymph node dissection in bladder cancer? Is it necessary also to remove bilateral common iliac lymph nodes? Some surgeons start from the aortic bifurcation and perform an extensive lymphadenectomy, skeletonizing the common, external, and interal iliac vessels circumferentially; others consider a limited dissection, below the iliac bifurcation, to suffice. The present authors perform pelvic lymph node dissection including the common iliac lymph nodes. In some cases only the common iliac nodes have proved positive, the external and internal iliac and obturator nodes all being negative.[6] Furthermore, including the common iliac lymph nodes has little effect on the surgical time, the invasiveness to the patient or the postoperative morbidity; the extensive lymphadenectomy is therefore desirable, in the authors' opinion.

Can pelvic lymph node dissection actually improve patient survival? Randomized trials are essential to obtain a clear-cut conclusion but, as yet, have not been carried out. According to the authors' data published in 1978 (i.e. data obtained from the authors' hospital at a time when pelvic lymph node dissection was seldom performed during total cystectomy), the 5-year survival rate was 82% for T_1 and T_2 cases, and only 9% for T_3 and T_4 cases.[7] In comparison to current results obtained with node dissection, high-stage tumours had a very poor prognosis, although the prognosis for low-stage tumours was similar in both sets of results. Despite these data referring to historical controls, and the total number of patients undergoing cystectomy being very small (25 cases), it would appear that node dissection is beneficial in cases of high-stage tumours.

One patient seen by the authors underwent total cystectomy, pelvic lymphadenectomy and ileal conduit for bladder cancer in 1978. The tumour was transitional cell carcinoma (grade 3, pT_3). Of four left internal iliac nodes removed, two contained cancer cells. The patient was followed without chemotherapy or irradiation and is now disease free. This case suggests that complete cure by total cystectomy combined with pelvic node dissection is theoretically possible if the metastases are confined to the lymph nodes and the lymph nodes affected by tumour are removed completely. In invasive bladder cancer, however, vascular invasion by the tumour cells is often seen. The therapeutic effects of pelvic lymph node dissection are therefore limited in invasive bladder cancer that can be regarded as a systemic disease. Pelvic lymph node dissection is theoretically of benefit to only a small proportion of patients whose nodal lesion is completely removed when metastasis is restricted to the pelvic nodes.

Neoadjuvant and adjuvant chemotherapies

To overcome the limitations of lymph node dissection, neoadjuvant or adjuvant chemotherapy has been developed. The effectiveness of these therapies in treating invasive bladder cancer has been demonstrated by many reports.[8–10] Some investigators, however, are sceptical about the efficacy of such treatment.[11–13] Although systemic chemotherapy has produced excellent results in patients with advanced bladder cancer, randomized trials have not yet conclusively demonstrated the improvement of survival to date. Whether these chemotherapies are really effective and, if so, which is the method of choice, remains open to debate.

With regard to MVAC, a representative chemotherapy regimen using methotrexate, vinblastine, Adriamycin (doxorubicin) and cisplatin, a group study in Japan showed that the incidence of major side effects was 85% for bone marrow suppression, 19% for sepsis following leucopenia and 41% for stomatitis.[14,15] Such side effects of MVAC therapy must give rise to concern.

Table 6.2 gives an example of the cost of MVAC therapy. In Japan, two cycles of MVAC therapy usually cost about US$20 000, including the expenses of medicines, hospitalization, examinations and granulocyte colony stimulating factor (GCSF) that is usually needed for the treatment of leucopenia following MVAC therapy. As mentioned above, systemic chemotherapy for invasive bladder cancer is not yet an established mode of treatment; it is indicated in carefully selected cases only, because of its toxicity and expense, the delay in surgery (neoadjuvant) and the long hospital stay.

Procedure	Cost	
	Japanese yen	American dollars
Chemotherapy[†]	455 100	4 551
Hospitalization (30 days)	342 480	3 425
Labo. examination	53 000	530
Other[‡]	151 950	1 520
Total	1 002 530	10 026

[†]Total cost of two cycles: ¥2 005 060 or US$20 052
[‡]Including GCSF, diuretic and antibiotics.
*Endoscopy, cytology, image diagnosis, etc.

Table 6.2. Cost of one cycle* of MVAC in a 40-year-old female with advanced bladder cancer

Laparoscopic lymph node dissection

The use of laparoscopic pelvic lymph node dissection (LPLND) for staging in prostate cancer has increased sharply in recent years, because it has been shown to be a minimally invasive procedure with excellent diagnostic value and has become an established technique in prostate cancer,[16] although not in bladder cancer. This is because the therapeutic regimen for bladder cancer needs to be less frequently modified than that for prostate cancer, even when LPLND finds small lymph node metastases that cannot be detected by preoperative CT scan.

With regard to the possible roles of LPLND in bladder cancer,[17–19] if total or partial cystectomy can be performed easily by laparoscopic surgery, LPLND will probably become used extensively in bladder cancer. It would then be indicated for the following cases of bladder cancer: (1) patients with pelvic tumours that cannot be biopsied under the guidance of ultrasound or CT, but in which a biopsy is necessary; (2) patients who refuse open surgery but in whom staging of the disease is necessary; (3) patients who are clinically suspected of having metastases that cannot be detected by imaging diagnosis and who require an examination to determine whether or not metastases are present; and (4) patients for whom the necessity of neoadjuvant therapy has to be determined.

The basic strategy currently used by the author for the treatment of bladder cancer is shown in Table 6.3. After the radical cystectomy, upon detection of lymph node metastasis or vascular invasion adjuvant therapy is started using MVAC. All T_4 patients also receive preoperative systemic chemotherapy. A new protocol for the treatment of bladder cancer is now being developed (Table 6.4). According to this protocol, T_4 cases without clinically distant metastasis first receive LPLND to detect the presence or absence of metastases in the nodes. Patients can then be divided into two groups: (1) if frozen sections show the nodes to

---

1. CIS; TUR + BCG* → Radical cystex if advanced
2. pT_a, pT_1; TUR + BCG → Radical cystex if advanced
3. T_2, T_3; Radical cystex
4. T_4; Neoadjuvant chemotherapy + Radical cystex

Adjuvant chemotherapy follows cystex if pN+ or pV+

---

*BCG, Bacillus Calmette-Guérin

Table 6.3. Current treatment strategy in bladder cancer

---

1. T_4:
    LPLND $\rightarrow$ pN + $\rightarrow$ Neoadjuvant $\rightarrow$ Cystex
     pN $-$ $\rightarrow$ Cystex

2. Small and solitary T_2, T_3:
    LPLND $\rightarrow$ pN + $\rightarrow$ Neoadjuvant $\rightarrow$ Cystex
     pN $-$ $\rightarrow$ Bladder preservation
     (intra-arterial or systemic chemotherapy, aggressive TUR,
     partial cystex)

Adjuvant chemotherapy after cystex if pV+

Table 6.4. Laparoscopic pelvic lymph node dissection (LPLND): new protocol

be positive, the patients are treated by neoadjuvant chemotherapy, with subsequent total cystectomy if possible, (2) if the nodes are negative as assessed by frozen section, patients subsequently undergo total cystectomy. If this new protocol is put into effect, neoadjuvant chemotherapy, which is currently used in all T_4 cases, will be restricted to those in whom it is considered to be essential, thus freeing the remainder from the side effects and expense of neoadjuvant therapy. Furthermore, in cases of small and solitary T_{2-3} tumours with laparoscopically confirmed negative nodes, it seems preferable to consider bladder preservation using aggressive transurethral resection (TUR), partial cystectomy or intra-arterial instillation of antimitotic agents.

Conclusions

The most important role of pelvic lymph node dissection is in predicting the prognosis by the examination of nodes. LPLND will play an important part in a new treatment strategy for bladder cancer, in combination with surgery and adjuvant or neoadjuvant chemotherapy, bearing in mind the risk–benefits and cost–benefits.

References

1. Aso Y, Ushiyama T, Tajima A *et al.* Treatment of 256 cases with bladder tumors. Jpn J Urol 1989; 80: 74–81
2. Logothetis C J, Dexeus F H, Finn L *et al.* A prospective randomized trial comparing MVAC and CISCA chemotherapy for patients with metastatic urothelial tumors. J Clin Oncol 1990; 8: 1050–1055

3. Smith J A, Whitmore W F Jr. Regional lymph node metastasis from bladder cancer. J Urol 1981; 126: 591–593

4. Skinner D G. Management of invasive bladder cancer: a meticulous pelvic node dissection can make a difference. J Urol 1982; 128: 34–36

5. Lerner S P, Skinner D G, Lieskovsky G et al. The rationale for en bloc pelvic node dissection for bladder cancer patients with nodal metastases: long-term results. J Urol 1993; 149: 3758–3765

6. Tomioka S, Isaka S, Okano T et al. Lymph node metastasis in bladder cancer. Jpn J Urol 1994; 85: 489–494

7. Takayasu H, Ogawa A, Kitagawa R et al. Treatment of tumors of the urinary bladder. Jpn J Urol 1978; 69: 669–678

8. Skinner D G, Daniels J R, Russel C A et al. The role of adjuvant chemotherapy following cystectomy for invasive bladder cancer: a prospective comparative trial. J Urol 1991; 145: 459–467

9. Stockle M, Meyenburg W, Wellek S et al. Advanced bladder cancer (stage pT3b, pT4a, pN1 and pN2): improved survival after radical cystectomy and 3 cycles of chemotherapy. Results of a controlled prospective study. J Urol 1992; 148: 302–307

10. Sternberg C N, Yagoda A, Scher H I et al. M-VAC for advanced transitional cell carcinoma of the urothelium: efficacy and patterns of response. Cancer 1989; 64: 2448–2458

11. Rintala E, Hannisdahl E, Fosa S D et al. Neoadjuvant chemotherapy in bladder cancer; a randomized study; Nordic cystectomy trial 1. Scand J Urol Nephrol 1993; 27: 355–362

12. Wallace D M A, Raghaven D, Kelly K A et al. Neo-adjuvant (preemptive) cisplatin therapy in invasive transitional cell carcinoma of the bladder. Br J Urol 1991; 67: 477–482

13. Tannock L, Gospodarowicz M, Connolly J et al. M-VAC (methotrexate, vinblastine, doxorubicin and cisplatin) chemotherapy for invasive transitional cell carcinoma: the Princess Margaret Hospital experience. J Urol 1989; 142: 289–292

14. Kotake T. Chemotherapy of invasive bladder cancer. Jpn J Cancer Chemother 1991; 18: 2375–2382

15. Kotake T, Niijima T, Akaza H et al. Evaluation of systemic chemotherapy with methotrexate, vinblastine, adriamycin, and cisplatin for bladder cancer. Cancer Chemother Pharmacol 1992; 30(suppl): S85–S89

16. Tajima A, Ueki, T. Laparoscopic pelvic lymph node dissection. Jpn J Endourol ESWL 1994; 7: 16–18

17. Roja C, Minguez J M, Blas M et al. Pelvic laparoscopic lymphadenectomy: a new option for staging bladder cancer. In: Villavicencio H, Fair W (eds) Evaluation of chemotherapy in bladder cancer. London: Churchill Livingstone, 1992: 79–89

18. Mazeman E, Wurtz A, Gilliot P et al. Extraperitoneal pelvioscopy in lymph node staging of bladder and prostate cancer. J Urol 1992; 147: 366–370

19. Rukstalis D B, Gerber G S, Vogelzang N J et al. Laparoscopic pelvic lymph node dissection: a review of 103 consecutive cases. J Urol 1994; 151: 670–674

Radical cystectomy and pelvic lymph node dissection in lymph-node-positive bladder cancer

7

J. E. Altwein

Introduction

The age-adjusted incidence per 100 000 person-years in bladder cancer has risen by 11% since 1975 to reach 32.3 in White American males. The mortality rate per 100 000 person-years (age-adjusted), however, has fallen since 1975 by 19.4% to a value of 5.8 in 1991.[1] The 5-year survival rates adjusted from normal life expectancy for patients with bladder cancer in the United States were 47% for White and 34% for Black Americans treated for regional disease, i.e. the majority will have positive lymph nodes (Fig. 7.1).[2] A population-based study from a Swiss canton demonstrated that the risk of infiltrating bladder cancer, which includes node-positive disease, is elevated in patients with superficial carcinoma of the urinary bladder.[3] The standardized incidence ratios were 48.2 for females and 15.6 for males. These ratios were highest between 1 and 4 years following registration of superficial cancer.

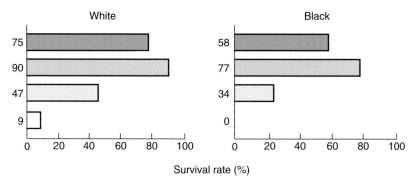

Figure 7.1. Five-year survival rates for (left) White and (right) Black patients with bladder cancer in the USA, diagnosed from 1983 to 1987. From top to bottom, histograms represent all stages, localized, regional and distant.

In patients subjected to cystectomy, invasion of the regional lymph nodes has long been recognized as the most important prognostic factor; in fact, all 23 patients with lymph node metastases at the time of cystectomy died within 3 years in this study from Bern.[4] In a similar observation involving 32 patients with cystectomy and pelvic lymph node dissection, the median survival was 13 months.[5] In a more recent study the covariables sex, grade, P category, N category, chemotherapy, radiotherapy, intravesical therapy and initial tumour stage were analysed by a multivariate study, which showed that the P category (confined to bladder versus not confined) and N category were the only significant covariables predicting long-term and disease-free survival.[6] In contradistinction to carcinoma of the prostate, patients with infiltrating and usually node-positive bladder cancer die from this specific cause.[7]

Diagnosis of lymph node metastases

The likelihood of lymph node metastases can be deduced from the grade and stage; this information is helpful in determining which patient needs an additional imaging study. In a retrospective analysis by Jacobi et al.,[8] none of the G_1 bladder tumours had lymph node metastases, all three G_2 were PN_1 and, of 16 G_3, six were PN_1, four PN_2, four PN_3 and two PN_4. The clinical stage of the primary tumour is correlated as follows: T_{is}, 0%; T_1, 5%; T_2, 13%; T_3, 18% and T_4, 44%.[9] The same is true for the P stage (Table 7.1). Imaging studies have been validated for their efficacy in distinguishing between intravesical and extravesical disease. See et al.[15] have compiled studies that compared computed tomography (CT) versus magnetic resonance imaging (MRI) versus ultrasound (US), and found

Series		Pa/Pis					
Ref. no.*	Year	P_1	P_2	$P_{2/3a}$	P_{3a}	P_{3b}	P_4
10	1979	0	–	18	–	30	50
4	1982	–	–	–	10	30	40
11	1985	0	6		30	–	59
12	1987	0	–	13	–	27	–
13	1988	5	30		31	64	50
14	1992	4	20		24	42	45

* As in reference list

Table 7.1. Incidence (%) of pelvic nodal metastases from bladder cancer according to pathological tumour stage

that the average sensitivity of CT in identifying extravesical tumour extent (stage T_{3b} or greater) is 70% versus 73% for MRI versus 60% for US (Fig. 7.2). The specificity is superior and is rated at 81% for CT, 84% for MRI and even 95% for US; however, there is still an understaging of 17% and an overstaging of 18% on average.[15]

In determining the nodal status in bladder cancer, the average sensitivity of CT is just 48%, but the specificity is 94% (Fig. 7.3). The main problem is the 52% understaging rate. The compiled figures for MRI to determine the nodal status are in the same range.[15] Invasive, laparascopic staging of the pelvic lymph nodes has never gained popularity, in contrast to prostate cancer, although it could be argued that if there is histological proof of positive lymph nodes, neoadjuvant chemotherapy could be started. In essence, imaging studies have a low sensitivity in detecting nodal metastases, which leads to the high rate of understaging; therefore, in the presence of high-grade and extravesical disease, negative imaging studies would be suspect.

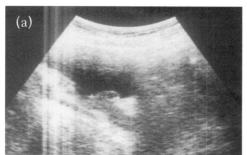
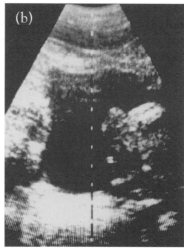

Figure 7.2. Ultrasound appearance of an infiltrating bladder cancer: (a) tumour in the left ureteral orifice; (b) T_{4a}-tumour in the left half of the bladder.

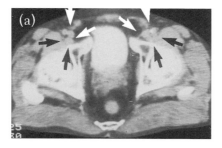
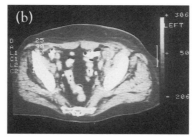

Figure 7.3. CT demonstrating (a) N_0 and (b) N_2 bladder tumour.

Technical considerations

In a number of institutions, cystectomy has not been carried out when positive lymph nodes were demonstrated during surgery.[4] This attitude is based on the conviction that the presence of lymph node metastases indicates the presence of systemic tumour that is not amenable to surgery. Jacobi et al.[8] have not shared this view and have demonstrated a difference in prognosis in patients subjected to radical cystectomy when the lymph nodes are removed at the same time; they showed that the 5-year survival rate reached 65% as opposed to 33% without pelvic lymphadenectomy. However, the lymphadenectomy group may be biased due to stage migration, case selection and — last but not least — operative technique. Nevertheless, 19 of 97 patients with lymphadenectomy and positive nodes are included in the 5-year survival calculation (Table 7.2).

The technique of pelvic lymphadenectomy in conjunction with radical cystectomy has been described in detail by Skinner;[20] thus, brief comments on technical niceties should suffice here. In the author's department, lymphadenectomy starts with the removal of Rosenmüller's lymph node medial to the external iliac artery at the femoral canal. Draining lymphatic vessels are secured with small, medium or large titanium haemoclips, in order not to impair follow-up by CT. In conjunction with removal of the obturator nodes, the inferior vesical artery is ligated peripherally and centrally clipped and cut. The second pedicle is secured in a similar manner when the lymph node dissection reaches the hypogastric trunk; the superior vesical artery is included.

| Series | | No. of | 5-year survival rate (%) for pathological stage | | | | |
Ref. no.*	Year	patients	P_0/P_1 cis	P_2	P_{3a}	P_{3b}	P_4 or N+
16	1964	61	–	50	16	12	–
4	1982	150	48	36	23	38	0
8	1983	153	52	41	39	28	–
17	1987	52	–	50	16	12	–
18	1981	58	71	88	57	40	29
19	1984	197	75	64	44		36
13	1988	189	83	83	69	29	27

* As in reference list.

Table 7.2. Therapeutic results of radical cystectomy for invasive bladder cancer

Irrespective of the type of diversion, the author attempts to preserve the peritoneum, whenever feasible. An exception is the pars afixa overlying the bladder dome. When the lateral peritoneum has been defatted downwards to the rectovesical pouch, the ureter is clipped and divided and a segment is sent for frozen section to avoid retention of carcinoma in situ. Giant histological sections have shown that the invasion of the mural lymphatic vessels is very closely related to the depth of infiltration of the primary neoplasm.[21] The extensive lymphatic network drains into large collecting trunks that are organized around three main regions, involving the trigone and posterior and anterior bladder walls. Between these collecting trunks, small perivesical lymph nodes are noted.[14] Smith et al.[9] noted that the obturator (74%), external iliac (65%) and common iliac nodes (19%) are most commonly involved; however, the latter is, always in the presence of ispilateral distal node involvement. Wishnow et al.[12] noted that unsuspected lymph node metastases were detected only on the same side as the bladder cancer, and pointed out that 80% of the unsuspected nodes were below the iliac bifurcation. This resulted in the widely held European opinion that no patient with nodes above the iliac bifurcation can be saved. Accordingly, in Europe the bifurcation has very often been considered to be at least the upper limit of nodal dissection, whereas in the American literature the nodes from the distal common iliac artery are included.[6,22] The nodes are subjected to pathological examination according to location, whereas the perivesical nodes are left with the cystectomy specimen (Fig. 7.4).

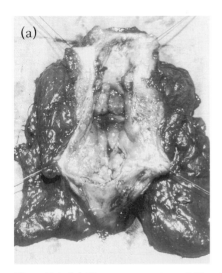
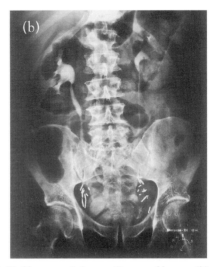

Figure 7.4. (a) Cystectomy specimen (pT_{3b} pN_1 bladder cancer) from a 59-year-old man; (b) IVP after cystectomy and pelvic lymphadenectomy (same patient as in Fig. 4a)

Complications of pelvic lymph node dissection

Although pelvic lymph node dissection is not completely separable from the complications of cystectomy, there are distinct undesirable side effects related to this additional procedure. The complication rate for cystectomy varies from 14 to 81%,[23] depending upon the accuracy of reporting. Directly related to pelvic lymphadenectomy are lymphocoele, lymphatic fistula, lymphoedema, arterial erosion and even pulmonary embolism. The latter is in the range of 2%, but must such patients die because of this side effect?[23,24] In addition, 'milder degrees of dependent oedema involving the legs and external genitalia were noted in many patients. Most responded well to the administration of diuretics, the use of TED stockings and the passage of time. Five per cent of our cases had oedema of a severe degree and in 4% it proved refractory to all treatment'.[24]

Outcome of cystectomy and lymphadenectomy

The stage-related 5-year survival rate for radical cystectomy varies considerably. It is particularly interesting when studying separately the survival rate of patients with positive lymph nodes (Table 7.3), which range from 0 to 36%. It is of note, however, that survival is usually not

Series		Percentage node positive	No. of N+ patients	5-year survival (%)
Ref. no.*	Year			
25	1962	20	46	4
26	1973	NS†	35	17
27	1973	20	64	8
28	1976	18	24	26
29	1980	15	26	4
9	1981	20	134	7
30	1982	24	36	36
4	1982	NS	23	0
22	1985	NS	57	10
11	1985	29	58	0–6
31	1988	NS	21	24 (> 40 months)
32	1991	15	42	19
14	1992	22	132	29
6	1994	NS	149	29

*As in reference list
†Not stated

Table 7.3. Five-year survival rate following radical cystectomy and pelvic lymphadenectomy in patients with pathological nodal metastases from bladder cancer

related to surgery alone: in the older literature, survival is related to the N stage (Fig. 7.5). Recently, Vieweg et al.[6] showed that the N category was significantly associated with disease-free survival. Median times to recurrence were 8.6 ± 2.9 months for pN_1, 7.9 ± 1.1 for pN_2 and 2.5 ± 1.7 for pN_3 tumours. The relapse-free survival at 6, 12 and 24 months, respectively, was 51.7% ± 9.3, 34.5% ± 8.5 and 10.3% ± 5.7 for pN_1; 51.0% ± 7.1; 38.8% ± 7.0 and 14.2% ± 5.0 for pN_2; and 20% ± 12.6 at 6 months for pN_3. Lerner et al.[14] noted, in 84 patients with one to five positive pelvic lymph nodes, a 5-year survival rate of 35 ± 11% and a 10-year survival rate of 24 ± 11%, as opposed to 17 ± 12% (at 5 and 10 years) for 48 patients with six or more positive lymph nodes. Basically, the correlation of the extent of nodal involvement being reported as the pN stage, the percentage of positive nodes or the absolute number of positive nodes to survival or the time to progression simply indicates that the bladder cancer was diagnosed at different timepoints during its evolution.

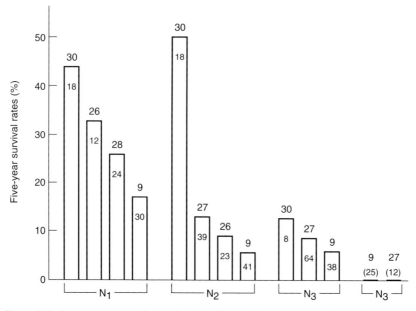

Figure 7.5. Cystectomy ± irradiation for pN+ disease: 5-year survival. Numerals surmounting columns refer to listed references; numerals within columns (or in parentheses) refer to numbers of patients.

Neoadjuvant and adjuvant therapy

Neoadjuvant chemotherapy has the advantage that the response to such therapy can be determined by pathological examination. This issue has been extensively discussed recently,[33] so only a few aspects are reiterated here. Altogether, five phase III studies of neoadjuvant chemotherapy have been completed. The design of these five studies involved radical cystectomy versus cisplatin before radical cystectomy (CUETO),[33] methotrexate versus radiotherapy and eventually salvage cystectomy (United Kingdom Cooperative Urological Cancer Group),[34] cisplatin versus radiotherapy (West Midland Urological Research Group),[35] cisplatin versus radiotherapy (Australian Bladder Cancer Study Group),[36] and cisplatin plus doxorubicin versus radiotherapy group cystectomy (Nordic Cooperative Bladder Cancer Study Group).[37]

Some of these neoadjuvant chemotherapy studies had accrual problems because of the subsequent availability of MVAC [methotrexate, vinblastine, Adriamycin (doxorubicin) and cisplatin] therapy. In the CUETO protocol, 79% of the patients allocated to cisplatin completed the cycles without modification and 87% eventually underwent cystectomy. It is of note, however, that in the Shearer study 60% of patients did not receive the planned maintenance chemotherapy. All five neoadjuvant studies have been subjected to meta-analysis after a median follow-up of approximately 3 years, and no survival advantage was found for patients receiving chemotherapy. The only prognostic factor for which there was evidence of a differential treatment effect across groups was age. Altogether, the results of neoadjuvant chemotherapy suggest that one of the more important objectives of neoadjuvant chemotherapy studies should be the effect on the primary lesion, as stated at the beginning of this section. On examining the results in patients with node-positive disease in the CUETO study (Table 7.4), no advantage of neoadjuvant chemotherapy can be detected. A problem independent of neoadjuvant chemotherapy is, however, the postoperative mortality.

One statistical problem in all five studies of neoadjuvant chemotherapy is the small sample size. To detect an absolute improvement of 10% in survival, 900 patients should be followed, which is the target of two ongoing trials of the EORTC and the British MRC study with CMV. Even if there were a small survival benefit or a benefit in time to progression attributable to preoperative chemotherapy, the problem of patient tolerance is of serious concern, particularly as the number of patients of node-positive bladder cancer represent a worst-case selection who barely tolerate cystectomy alone, and the median survival for this group is 11.9 ± 5.1 months.[6]

Treatment	Tumour	No. of patients	Survival (%)	Cancer deaths (%)	Postop. deaths (%)
Control	pN_0	36	49.9	2.5	13.8
	pN_1	6	33.3	16.6	50.0
	pN_{2-4}	13	12.5	75.0	0.0
Cisplatin (X3)	pN_0	38	47.2	39.5	13.1
	pN_1	10	40.0	40.0	10.0
	pN_{2-4}	6	0.0	83.3	0.0

*From CUETO 84005.[33]

*Table 7.4. Neoadjuvant cisplastin before cystectomy in 109 patients with bladder cancer**

Adjuvant chemotherapy

Adjuvant chemotherapy has the advantage that the pathological stage of the disease at the time of surgery is known precisely. Proponents see potential risks associated with delaying primary surgery when subjecting the patient to any preoperative treatment and with exposure to the toxicity of chemotherapy, particularly multiple chemotherapy. In contrast to neoadjuvant therapy, adjuvant therapy has the disadvantage of lacking proof of the response. Logothetis et al.[38] noted that adjuvant CISCA benefited patients with node-positive disease; subsequently, two prospective phase III trials demonstrated an advantage of adjuvant chemotherapy. Skinner et al.[39] performed a randomized trial after radical cystectomy plus pelvic lymphadenectomy in 91 patients receiving four cycles of CISCA versus observation; in 36% of these 91 patients there were positive lymph nodes. In patients with one positive lymph node (of whom 10 were observed and seven received CISCA), the time to progression and the survival was significantly improved for the chemotherapy patients; this advantage was lost in patients with two or more positive nodes. The study has been severely criticized for methodological errors.[36] Stöckle et al.[40] randomized patients after cystectomy to adjuvant M-VEC or MVAC; the number of lymph nodes involved ranged from none to 10 in the 26 chemotherapy patients (median 1.0) versus none to three in the 23 control patients (median 1.0). There was a significant decrease in the risk of tumour recurrence after adjuvant chemotherapy. The number of lymph nodes involved was also of prognostic significance, an observation which is in keeping with Skinner's study.

Conclusions

Pelvic lymphadenectomy allows for better staging, but only the occasional patient with microscopic node involvement or solitary nodes may benefit from this approach. More aggressive lymphadenectomy, dissecting the nodes up to the aortic bifurcation, does not necessarily translate to an improved survival.

Multiple neoadjuvant chemotherapy has been tried in patients with node-positive disease, but practical problems such as reduced tolerance of surgery may interfere with any possible benefit. For the surgeon, adjuvant chemotherapy appears to have advantages. A review of new agents for use in advanced bladder cancer had recently been published.[41]

References

1. Devesa S S, Blot W J, Stone B J, Miller B A. Recent cancer trends in the United States. J Natl Cancer Inst 1995; 87: 175–182
2. Boring C C, Squires T S, Tong T, Cancer statistics, 1993. CA 1993; 43: 7–26
3. Levi F, La Vecchia C, Randimbison L, Franceschi S. Incidence of infiltrating cancer following superficial bladder carcinoma. Int J Cancer 1993; 55: 419–421
4. Studer U E, Imhof F, Zingg E J, Faktoren, welche die Überlebensrate nach radikaler Zystektomie bestimmen. Helv Chir Acta 1982; 49: 375–379
5. Breuel F, Altwein J E, Schneider W, Stellenwert der pelvinen Lymphknotendissektion im Rahmen der erweiterten radikalen Zystektomie beim Blasenkarzinom. Verh Dtsch Ges Urol 1986; 38: 40–41
6. Vieweg J, Whitmore W F Jr. Herr H W et al. The role of pelvic lymphadenectomy and radical cystectomy for lymph node positive bladder cancer. The Memorial Sloan-Kettering Cancer Center experience. Cancer 1994; 72: 1099–1105
7. Hellsten S, Glifberg I, Lindholm CE, Telhammer E. Therapy of bladder carcinoma. Scand J Urol Nephrol 1981; 15: 115–120
8. Jacobi G H, Klippel K F, Hohenfellner R, 15 Jahre Erfahrung mit der radikalen Zystektomie ohne präoperative Radiotherapie beim Harnblasenkarzinom. Aktuel Urol 1983; 14: 63–69
9. Smith J A Jr. Whitmore W F Jr. Regional lymph node metastasis from bladder cancer. J Urol 1981; 126: 591–593
10. Prout G R Jr, Griffin P P, Shipley W U. Bladder carcinoma as a systemic disease. Cancer 1979; 43: 2532
11. Giuliani L, Giberti C, Martorana G et al. Results of radical cystectomy for primary bladder cancer: retrospective study of more than 200 cases. Urology 1985; 26: 243
12. Wishnow K I, Tenney T M. Will Rogers and the results of radical cystectomy for invasive bladder cancer. Urol Clin North Am 1991; 18: 529
13. Skinner D G, Liesovsky G. Management of invasive and high-grade bladder cancer. In Skinner D G, Lieskovsky G (eds) Diagnosis and management of genitourinary cancer. Philadelphia: Saunders, 1988; 295–312

14. Lerner S P, Skinner E, Skinner D G. Radical cystectomy in regionally advanced bladder cancer. Urol Clin North Am 1992; 19: 713–723

15. See W, Fuller W. Staging of advanced bladder cancer. Urol Clin North Am 1992; 19: 663–683

16. Jewett H J, Strong G H. Infiltrating carcinoma of the bladder: relation of depth of penetration of the bladder wall to incidence of local extension and metastases. J Urol 1946; 55: 366

17. Pearse H D, Reed R R, Hodges C V. Radical cystectomy for bladder cancer. J Urol 1978; 119: 216

18. Mathur V K, Krahn H P, Ramsey E W. Total cystectomy for bladder cancer. J Urol 1981; 125: 784–786

19. Skinner D G, Lieskovsky G. Contemporary cystectomy with pelvic node dissection compared to preoperative radiation therapy plus cystectomy in the management of invasive bladder cancer. J Urol 1984; 131: 1069

20. Skinner D G. The craft of urologic surgery. Urol Clin North Am 1981; 8: 353–366

21. Soto E A, Friedell G H, Tretman A J. Bladder cancer as seen in giant histologic sections. Cancer 1977; 39: 447–455

22. Zincke H, Patterson D E, Utz D C, Benson R C Jr. Pelvic lymphadenectomy and radical cystectomy for transitional cell carcinoma of the bladder with pelvic nodal disease. Br J Urol 1985; 57: 156–159

23. Kutscher H A, Leadbetter G W Jr, Vinson R K. Survival after radical cystectomy for invasive transitional cell carcinoma of bladder. Urology 1981; 17: 231–234

24. Thomas D M, Riddle P R. Morbidity and mortality in 100 consecutive radical cystectomies. Br J Urol 1982; 54: 716–719

25. Vieweg J, Whitmore W F, Herr H W, Sogani P C, Russo P, Sheinfeld J, Fair W R. The role of pelvic lymphadenectomy and radical cystectomy for lymph node positive bladder cancer. Cancer 1994; 73: 3020–3028

26. Dretler S P, Ragsdale B D, Leadbetter W F. The value of pelvic lymphadenectomy in the surgical treatment of bladder cancer. J Urol 1973; 109: 414

27. Laplante M, Brice M II. The upper limits of hopeful application of radical cystectomy for vesical carcinoma: does nodal metastasis always indicate incurability? J Urol 1973; 109: 261

28. Reid E C, Oliver J A, Fishman I J. Preoperative irradiation and cystectomy in 135 cases of bladder cancer. Urology 1976; 8: 247

29. Bredael J J, Croker B P, Glenn J F. The curability of invasive bladder cancer treated by radical cystoprostatectomy. Eur Urol 1980; 6: 206

30. Skinner D G. Management of invasive bladder cancer: a meticulous pelvic node dissection can make a difference. J Urol 1982; 128: 34

31. Grossman H B, Konnak J W. Is radical cystectomy indicated in patients with regional lymphatic metastases? Urology 1988; 31: 214

32. Roehrborn C G, Sagalowsky A I, Peters P C. Longterm patient survival after cystectomy for regional metastatic transitional cell carcinoma of the bladder. J Urol 1991; 146: 36

33. Martinez-Pineiro J A, Martin M G, Arocena F et al. Neoadjuvant cisplatin chemotherapy before radical cystectomy in invasive transitional cell carcinoma of the bladder: a prospective randomized phase III study. J Urol 1995; 153: 964–73

34. Shearer R J, Chilvers C F, Bloom H J et al. Adjuvant chemotherapy in t_3 carcinoma of the bladder. A prospective trial: preliminary report. Br J Urol 1988; 62: 558

35. Wallace D M A, Raghavan D, Kelly K A *et al*. Neoadjuvant (pre-emptive) cisplatin therapy in invasive transitional cell carcinoma of the bladder. Br J Urol 1991; 67: 608–615

36. Raghavan D. Neoadjuvant and classic adjuvant chemotherapy for bladder cancer. Curr Opin Urol 1991; 1: 53

37. Rintala E, Hannisdahl E, Hellsten S *et al*. Neoadjuvant chemotherapy and radiotherapy prior to cystectomy of locally advanced bladder cancer. In: Villavicencio H, Fair W R (eds) Evaluation of chemotherapy in bladder cancer. Edinburgh: Churchill Livingstone, 1992; 17: 197–211

38. Logothetis C J, Johnson D E, Chong C *et al*. Adjuvant cyclophosphamide, doxorubicin, and cisplatin chemotherapy for bladder cancer: an update. J Clin Oncol 1988; 6: 1590+

39. Skinner D G, Daniels J R, Russell D A *et al*. The role of adjuvant chemotherapy following cystectomy for invasive bladder cancer. A prospective comparative trial. J Urol 1991; 145: 459–476

40. Stöckle M, Meyenburg W, Wellek S *et al*. Advanced bladder cancer (stages pT3b, pT4a, pN1 and pN2): improved survival after radical cystectomy and 3 adjuvant cycles of chemotherapy. Results of a controlled prospective study. J Urol 1992; 148: 302–307

41. Roth B J, Bajaorin D F, Advanced bladder cancer: the need to identify new agents in the post-M-VAC (methotrexate, vinblastine, doxorubicin and cisplatin) world. J Urol 1995; 153: 894–900

Prostate

IV

Alternative surgical techniques to pelvic lymphadenectomy in the staging of prostate cancer

8

R. O. Parra   J. M. Cummings
E. Mazeman

Introduction

Recent advances in the early detection of prostate cancer, such as widespread implementation of serum prostate-specific antigen (PSA) testing, together with transrectal ultrasound-guided prostatic biopsies, have undoubtedly increased the number of (potentially curable) men diagnosed with this disease. Concurrently, the number of patients undergoing surgical treatment by radical prostatectomy has also taken an upturn. A distinct adverse prognostic factor in men with prostate cancer is the presence of lymph node metastases. Unfortunately, at present there is no non-invasive imaging modality that can reliably identify those individuals afflicted with nodal involvement. Surgical staging by way of a pelvic lymph node dissection therefore remains the mainstay of the diagnosis of nodal metastases in patients undergoing definitive treatment for clinically localized prostatic carcinoma. Open pelvic lymphadenectomy, however, is not devoid of complications: a review of the literature reveals a 29% incidence of postoperative complications.[1] Together with these associated adverse events, the introduction of significant technical advances in endoscopic instrumentation has inspired a search for a less invasive approach to the staging of the pelvic lymph nodes, leading to the development and application of several novel techniques with the common objective of eliminating a laparotomy incision while reducing morbidity and convalescence of those patients with nodal metastases. This review puts such alternative methods into perspective and delineates their role in the staging of the patient with prostate cancer.

Pelvioscopic lymphadenectomy

Hald first described extraperitoneal pelvioscopy for staging lower urinary tract tumours in 1980, using a technique advocated by Bartel who modified an earlier method of Maasen.[2,3] The technique was streamlined by Mazeman, who reported its use in 101 patients, 36 of whom had prostate cancer with the remainder having carcinoma of the bladder.[4] In that study, there were only two false-negative pelvioscopic lymph node dissections in the prostate cancer group, giving a reliability of 94%. The results for pelvioscopy in the bladder cancer group were similar, as were the findings of Oveson et al. in another study using a similar pelvioscopic technique for detection of disseminated bladder neoplasm.[5] Furthermore, the technique has been modified to explore the lumbar retroperitoneal space to aid in the diagnosis of retroperitoneal masses such as those caused by Hodgkin's disease or lymphomas.[6]

The technique described uses a modified mediastinoscope through which instruments are passed. An incision of 3–4 cm is made approximately two fingerbreadths above and medial to the inguinal ligament. After the fascia has been incised, the muscle fibres are split and blunt finger dissection is used to separate the underlying peritoneum from the pelvic sidewall. The external iliac vessels are palpated and a small retractor is placed to displace their peritoneal contents. The pelvioscope is gently inserted and inspection of the area is carried out with excision of the nodes.

The future of this procedure may lie in improved technology for extraperitoneal node dissection, such as the use of balloon dilation to create space needed for the procedure,[7] or specialized endoscopic equipment to expose the area of interest.[8] Others have reported the use of CO_2 insufflation with standard laparoscopic equipment and ports to achieve lymphadenectomy.[9] Certainly, avoidance of the transperitoneal route may make the procedure safer if further studies confirm equivalency of efficacy.

Laparoscopic lymphadenectomy

The ability to gain access to the lymphatic drainage of the prostate gland in a truly minimally invasive fashion may well have revolutionized the treatment of prostatic carcinoma. Endoscopic node dissection gives the potential to stage disease accurately for non-surgical forms of therapy. It also has revived the radical perineal prostatectomy as a viable therapeutic alternative for cancer of the prostate.

Laparoscopy for pelvic lymphadenectomy was first described for cervical carcinoma in 1991.[10] In the same year, Schuessler reported on his initial experience in the use of laparoscopic pelvic node dissection (LPLND) for prostate cancer.[11] Since then, numerous papers have addressed the efficacy of LPLND, showing no difference in numbers of nodes harvested, as well as absence of retained nodes when LPLND is compared with standard open lymphadenectomy.[12–16] The morbidity of the procedure has also been extensively studied.[17,18]

The procedure involves placement of a laparoscopic camera through a small subumbilical incision into the peritoneal cavity. Additional working ports are placed in the right and left lower quadrants under vision to allow the introduction of dissecting instruments. After peritoneotomy over the iliac vessels, node dissection is performed. Nodal tissue is removed from the pubic ramus proximally to the bifurcation of the hypogastric and external iliac arteries followed by the obturator fossa. The procedure allows for easy access to both sides of the pelvis for a complete bilateral dissection.

The proper role of LPLND in the management of prostate cancer has yet to be finally determined. Its use as a minimally invasive staging modality prior to definitive radiation therapy has obvious appeal. To date, however, the combination of LPLND with radiotherapy has not been examined critically with regard to morbidity or results. Studies of this kind could also conceivably aid in the definition of the therapeutic role of radiation in prostate cancer, given the uncertainty of clinical staging found in most men treated in this manner.

Some studies have examined the proper place of LPLND in the surgical management of prostate carcinoma, particularly in conjunction with radical perineal prostatectomy.[19–22] This combination has been found to cause less morbidity than the standard retropubic approach and the length of the surgery has not been found to be excessive, even when including the time to shift patient positioning. In Parra's study,[21] a direct comparison was made between open node dissection plus retropubic approach versus LPLND plus retropubic approach, versus LPLND plus the perineal approach. Owing to decreased blood loss and hospital stay, it was concluded that the true value of LPLND was in combination with radical perineal prostatectomy. Again, however, there have not been any long-term studies showing the effectiveness of this combination of procedures in curing adenocarcinoma of the prostate, although one can infer from the effectiveness data of LPLND and the literature on the benefit of perineal prostatectomy[23,24] that it should be successful.

One final criticism of LPLND is that it may be associated with a higher complication rate than standard lymphadenectomy. The complication rate, as reported in both single-centre[18] and multicentre[17,25] trials, averages around 16%, which compares favourably with the complication rate reported in open procedures.[1] There does appear to be a steep learning curve that is difficult to conquer but, with the performance of multiple procedures, the number of complications decreases.[26]

Minilaparotomy

Reduction of the morbidity of formal laparotomy for lymphadenectomy while maintaining completeness of the procedure is the goal of the 'minilaparotomy' approach to the pelvic nodes. A method for this approach has been described by Steiner and Marshall.[27] They describe pelvic lymphadenectomy through a 6 cm lower abdominal incision. By manipulation of the incision and the skilful use of retractors they are able to expose the nodal package under direct vision and perform the dissection. In comparing this technique with a standard lymph node dissection, they found similar numbers of nodes retrieved by either method. There were no untoward events in the minilaparotomy group.

The advantages of the minilaparotomy procedure include a small incision, with resultant reduced morbidity if the nodes are positive and the patient does not go on to radical prostatectomy. It requires neither special expertise and/or training nor expensive equipment, as does laparoscopy for node dissection. The incision does, however, place this technique at a disadvantage if radical perineal prostatectomy is contemplated as the curative surgery for the prostatic carcinoma. Furthermore, there are no quantitative data at present as to reduction of postoperative pain in these patients as evidenced by a decrease in the amount of analgesics used. Although minilaparotomy has potential use in the area of prostate cancer staging, it awaits larger trials, perhaps in conjunction with perineal prostatectomy, before its real utility can be assessed.

Elimination of lymphadenectomy

As data concerning the predictive value for nodal metastases of such parameters as clinical stage, Gleason grade and serum PSA have accumulated, many have questioned the need for routine lymphadenectomy in men with prostate cancer. In studies correlating preoperative PSA levels with final pathological stage, elevations in PSA closely parallel increasing pathological stage.[28,29] In fact, in Lange's series, 59% of men with PSA above 10 had positive nodes or seminal vesicle involvement.[30] Parra[31] and Wolf[32] found that combining PSA, Gleason grade and clinical stage consistently predicted pathological stages. In a recent series of 1632 consecutive men undergoing radical prostatectomy, the probability of positive nodes was found to be less than 3.5% if the local clinical stage was T_1–T_{2b}, primary Gleason grade was 3 or less and the preoperative PSA was 10 or less.[33]

With the proliferation of these data, studies have ensued prospectively analysing performance of radical prostatectomy without node dissection in selected patients. A multicentre study presented this year showed no biochemical evidence of persistent or recurrent disease in a group of 24 men undergoing perineal prostatectomy alone.[34] The criteria for selection were PSA of less than 10, Gleason score of less than 7 and clinically organ-confined tumour. Although good results have been obtained thus far, follow-up is less than 2 years. Certainly, long-term follow-up is critical to determining if, in fact, this approach is sound.

Conclusion

Table 8.1 summarizes the advantages and disadvantages of each approach discussed. Clearly, the subject of lymphadenectomy in prostate cancer is one that is in flux, and the rise of minimally invasive methods of assessing the pelvic nodes gives urologists new food for thought on this topic. It appears that laparoscopic techniques are established as a viable method for lymph node dissection and are indicated when there is a high probability of metastases. Certainly, extraperitoneal pelvioscopy deserves consideration as a staging method that avoids the peritoneal contents while maintaining minimal invasiveness. The minilaparotomy may be

Technique	Advantages	Disadvantages
Pelvioscopy	Avoids peritoneal cavity; easier to learn	Exposure may be limited
Laparoscopy	Excellent exposure of pelvic nodes	Transperitoneal technique; steep learning curve
Minilaparotomy	Easiest to learn; standard OR equipment	Does have incision with retraction of muscles — potential for postoperative pain
No lymphadenectomy	No morbidity from lymph node dissection	Depending on selection criteria, some patients will have positive nodes

Table 8.1. Minimally invasive techniques to assess pelvic lymph nodes

equally useful for those lacking laparoscopic equipment or expertise. Finally, as more data accumulate, the ultimate question of the true need for lymphadenectomy may be answered for the improvement of patient care by the reduction of the morbidity induced by lymph node dissection itself. It is readily apparent that the real utility of these methods is in men at the extremes of tumour presentation. The authors' current recommendations for pelvic node assessment in localized prostate cancer are delineated in Figure 8.1.

Prostate Cancer Diagnosed

Clinical Staging
Gleason Score
PSA

Clinical Stage T_1–T_2	All others	Clinical Stage T_{2B-3} or greater
Gleason Score < 7	Patient preferences	Gleason Score ≥ 7
PSA < 10		PSA > 20

Radical perineal prostatectomy without lymphadenectomy	LPND and radical perineal prostatectomy	Standard open lymphadenectomy and radical retropubic prostatectomy	LPND
			negative nodes
			Radical perineal prostectomy

Figure 8.1. Current recommendations for assessment of pelvic nodes in localized prostate cancer.

References

1. McDowell G C, Johnson J W, Tenney D M, Johnson D E. Pelvic lymphadenectomy for staging clinically localized prostate cancer. Urology 1990; 25: 476
2. Hald T, Rasmussen F. Extraperitoneal pelvioscopy: a new aid in staging of lower urinary tract tumors. A preliminary report. J Urol 1980; 124: 245
3. Bartel M. Die retroperitoneoskopie: eine endoskopische methode zur inspektion und bioptischen untersuchung des retroperitonealen raumes. Zentralbl Chir 1969; 94: 377
4. Mazeman E, Wurtz A, Gilliot P, Biserte J. Extraperitoneal pelvioscopy in lymph node staging of bladder and prostatic cancer. J Urol 1992; 147: 366
5. Oveson H, Iversen P, Beier-Holgersen R et al. Extraperitoneal pelvioscopy in staging of bladder carcinoma and detection of pelvic lymph nodes metastasis. Scand J Urol Nephrol 1993; 27: 211
6. Mazeman E. Unpublished data, 1994
7. Masters J E, Fraundorfer M R, Gilling P J. Extraperitoneal laparoscopic pelvic lymph node dissection using the Gaur balloon technique. Br J Urol 1994; 74: 128
8. Etwaru D, Raboy A, Ferzli G, Albert P. Extraperitoneal endoscopic gasless pelvic lymph node dissection. J Laparoendosc Surg 1994; 4: 113

9. Villers A, Vannier J L, Abecassis R *et al.* Extraperitoneal endosurgical lymphadenectomy with insufflation in the staging of bladder and prostate cancer. J Endourol 1993; 7: 229

10. Querleu D, LeBlanc E, Castelain B. Laparoscopic lymphadenectomy in the staging of early carcinoma of the cervix. Am J Obstet Gynecol 1991; 164: 579

11. Schuessler W W, Vancaillie T G, Reich H, Griffith D P. Transperitoneal endosurgical lymphadenectomy in patients with localized prostate cancer. J Urol 1991; 145: 988

12. Parra R O, Andrus C H, Boullier J A. Staging laparoscopic pelvic lymph node dissection: comparison of results with open pelvic lymphadenectomy. J Urol 1992; 147: 875

13. Rioja Sanz C, Blas-Marin M, Rioja Sanz L. Laparoscopic pelvic lymphadenectomy in the staging of prostate cancer. Eur Urol 1993; 24: 19

14. Madsen M R, Holm-Nielsen A. Laparoscopic lymphadenectomy. Preliminary experience. Scand J Urol Nephrol 1993; 27: 215

15. Rukstalis D B, Gerber G S, Vogelzang N J *et al.* Laparoscopic pelvic lymph node dissection: a review of 103 consecutive cases. J Urol 1994; 151: 670

16. Kerbl K, Clayman R V, Petros J A *et al.* Staging pelvic lymphadenectomy for prostate cancer: a comparison of laparoscopic and open techniques. J Urol 1993; 150: 396

17. Kavoussi L R, Sosa E, Chandhoke P J *et al.* Complications of laparoscopic pelvic lymph node dissection. J Urol 1993; 149: 322

18. Parra R O, Hagood P G, Boullier J A *et al.* Complications of laparoscopic urologic surgery: experience at St Louis University. J Urol 1994; 151: 681

19. Levy D A, Resnick M I. Laparoscopic pelvic lymphadenectomy and radical perineal prostatectomy: a viable alternative to radical retropubic prostatectomy. J Urol 1994; 151: 905

20. Lerner S E, Fleischmann J, Taub H C *et al.* Combined laparoscopic pelvic lymph node dissection and modified Belt radical perineal prostatectomy for localized prostatic adenocarcinoma. Urology 1994; 43: 493

21. Parra R O, Boullier J A, Rauscher J A, Cummings J M. The value of laparoscopic lymphadenectomy in conjunction with a radical perineal or a retropubic prostatectomy. J Urol 1994; 151: 1599–1602

22. Thomas R, Steele R, Smith R, Brannan W. One-stage laparoscopic pelvic lymphadenectomy and radical perineal prostatectomy. J Urol 1994; 152: 1174

23. Paulson D F, Moul J W, Walther P J. Radical prostatectomy for clinical stage T1-2N0M0 prostatic adenocarcinoma: long-term results. J Urol 1990; 144: 1180

24. Thrasher J B, Paulson D F. Reappraisal of radical perineal prostatectomy. Eur Urol 1992; 22: 1

25. Kozminski M, Gomella L, Stone N *et al.* Laparoscopic urologic surgery: outcome assessment. J Urol 1992; 147: 245A

26. Lang G S, Ruckle H C, Hadley H R *et al.* One hundred consecutive laparoscopic pelvic lymph node dissections: comparing complications of the first 50 cases to the second 50 cases. Urology 1994; 44: 221

27. Steiner M S, Marshall F F. Mini-laparotomy staging pelvic lymphadenectomy (minilap): alternative to standard and laparoscopic pelvic lymphadenectomy. Urology 1993; 41: 201

28. Hudson M A, Bahnson R R, Catalona W J. Clinical use of prostate specific antigen in patients with prostate cancer. J Urol 1989; 142: 1011

29. Lange P H, Ercole C J, Lightner D J *et al.* The value of serum prostate specific antigen determination before and after radical prostatectomy. J Urol 1989; 141: 873

30. Lange P H. Prostate specific antigen for staging prior to surgery and for early detection of recurrence after surgery. Urol Clin North Am 1990; 17: 813

31. Parra R O, Andrus C H, Boullier J A. Staging laparoscopic pelvic lymph node dissection. Experience and indications. Arch Surg 1992; 127: 1294

32. Wolf J S, Shinohara K, Kerlikowske K M et al. Selection of patients for laparoscopic pelvic lymphadenectomy prior to radical prostatectomy: a decision analysis. Urology 1993; 42: 680

33. Bluestein D L, Bostwick D G, Bergstralh E J, Oesterling J E. Eliminating the need for bilateral pelvic lymphadenctomy in select patients with prostate cancer. J Urol 1994; 151: 1315

34. Isorna S, Parra R O, Garcia-Perez M et al. The radical perineal prostatectomy alone. Can we avoid the lymphadenectomy in the laparoscopic era? Programme of the Société Internationale D'Urologie 23rd Congress, 18–22 Sept 1994: 247 (abstr 624)

Role of laparoscopic pelvic lymphadenectomy in prostate cancer

9

C. Rioja Sanz   M. Blas Marin
C. Allepuz Losa   L. A. Rioja Sanz

Introduction

The improvement in diagnostic methods achieved in the last few years has permitted a greater approximation to the correct staging of pelvic neoplastic pathology in urology and specifically in prostate cancer. Prostate carcinoma is the fifth most frequently found cancer among males worldwide and has a greater frequency in industrialized countries.[1] It represents the second cause of mortality among males,[2] with a global rate of 22.6 per 100 000 inhabitants.[3] In Spain, it represents the third cause of death by neoplasia among males.[4] The probability of developing the disease in the Caucasian and Black races is 8.6 and 9.4%, respectively.[5] Knowledge of local node involvement is crucial in order to apply a correct therapeutic regimen and to determine the prognosis of the disease. Currently, there is a progressive diffusion of radical treatment (through surgery or radiotherapy) in patients with clinically localized prostate carcinoma where the impact of such therapy on control of the disease appears to be evident.[6–8] The principal problem concerns staging, as more than one-half of the patients have involvement outside the prostatic capsule at the time of diagnosis,[4,9] and have therefore only a small probability of their cancer being controlled by surgery or radiotherapy.

Diagnostic methodology is progressing in various directions, one of which is an attempt to specify node staging precisely in order to avoid aggressive treatment in patients where these techniques are of little benefit.[10]

That nodal involvement in prostatic cancer is one of the signs of a poor prognosis and that it is going to show the way unequivocally to survival in this disease in future is a fact and has been ratified by major series. It is also going to determine the subsequent therapeutic regimen.

The retrospective study performed by Gervasi[11] on a total of 511 patients with prostate carcinoma has demonstrated a greater risk for the development of metastases and death within 10 years with positive nodes, even in those with micrometastases in a single node. At present there is no non-invasive diagnostic method that detects the presence of adenopathy in prostate cancer with acceptable certainty. Ultrasonography permits only the recognition of large adenopathies in the pelvic region, and is therefore not a valid method. Lymphography, a method in use for more than 30 years, presents technical problems as it cannot consistently locate the hypogastric, presacral and obturator ganglia.[12] This, together with the important incidence of micrometastases accounts for the high rate of false negatives. False positives are produced in particular by the fatty substitution of nodal tissue in the elderly.[13] The association of fine-needle aspiration cytology (FNAC) decreases the rate of false positives but not the rate of false negatives, and is therefore not a completely accurate technique. Isotopic lymphography, using acid antiphosphate antibodies[14] or anti-prostate-specific antigen (anti-PSA) monoclonal antibodies tagged with iodine-25 (ref. 15) has opened a new field; it is too early, however, to evaluate its diagnostic accuracy. The value of CT is limited to providing information regarding nodal volume only, without distinguishing the intrinsic structure of the node; the determination of pathological size is controversial.[16] As with lymphography, the association of FNAC decreases the incidence of false positives. In general, CT is considered to have a sensitivity of 50–75%, a specificity of 80–100% and a diagnostic accuracy of 83–92%.[13,17,18] CT has advantages over the previously mentioned methods, but does not detect micrometastases. The role of magnetic resonance imaging (MRI) is similar to that of CT and offers a diagnostic accuracy of 83–89%.[19–22]

Once the limitations of the diagnostic imaging methods are accepted, and given the great interest in knowing the extent of nodal involvement, it must be recognized that lymphadenectomy is the most trustworthy technique to hand. Conventional surgical lymphadenectomy defines the state of the nodes but has the following disadvantages:

1. Elevated morbidity due to complications such as thromboembolism and lymphocoele. The series by Donohue[23] reflects up to 20% complications and Johnson[24] describes up to 22%.
2. High incidence of false negatives due to the limitations of the histopathological study of the fresh-frozen intraoperative specimens or due to an insufficient number of sections studied. The studies by Kramalowsky[25] and Epstein[26] confirmed this and reported a rate of

false negatives of approximately 27%. More recently, Hermansen and Whitmore[27] performed a study reviewing the most important series and obtained a 28.6% rate of false negatives.

3. There is an inevitable psychological impact of a laparotomy on the patient when the nodes are positive and it is not followed by radical surgery.

The adaptation of the extraperitoneal pelvioscopy performed by Bartel[28] in 1969 on the retroperitoneum was also performed by Hald and Rasmussen[29] starting in 1980, but was developed most by Mazeman,[30,31] beginning in 1985. Samples of the nodal tissue are taken from the iliac and obturator areas through two small abdominal incisions. This technique has the inconvenience of not obtaining a sufficient number of nodes and favouring the appearance of false negatives.

The known difficulty in detecting nodal involvement by non-invasive methods, as well as the 28.6% of false negatives in the intraoperative frozen biopsies, has encouraged the development of nodal biopsy using laparoscopic lymphadenectomy. This technique was described by Schuessler[32] in 1990 and performed by the authors' group in the same year.[33,34] It is a detailed and precise surgical technique that permits the total extraction of nodal tissue and is completely comparable to conventional open surgery. It does, however, offer advantages that can be summarized as follows:

1. It is a less aggressive method than open lymphadenectomy and has lower morbidity rates;
2. It avoids laparotomy in cases where there is nodal involvement;
3. It avoids false negatives from the frozen histopathological studies;
4. It avoids surgical procedures in cases of perineal prostatectomy;
5. It avoids laparotomy in patients treated with definitive radiotherapy.

To the above should be added the positive psychological acceptance by the patient and the almost 100% diagnostic accuracy. It is a technique that requires previous training, owing to its relative complexity; a steep and costly learning curve is therefore unavoidable. At present, pelvic laparoscopic lymphadenectomy is a real alternative to the traditional open surgical techniques, and constitutes the most important laparoscopic technique of our speciality.

Patients and results

Between November 1990 and February 1994 the authors performed laparoscopic pelvic lymphadenectomy in a total of 52 patients, detecting node involvement in 10 patients (19.23%). Node dissection is initiated on the side that suggests the greatest probability of infiltration,[35] or in the prostatic lobule involved according to the histopathological study, or the hardest node found in clinical exploration (if both are neoplastic). In this last case, some authors suggest that the dissection should be initiated on the side where the biopsy has shown a more unfavourable Gleason score.[36] If there are no specific differential data, the authors start the lymphadenectomy on the right side as it is a less complex dissection, for anatomical reasons.

The incidence by stage was of only one T_1 with node infiltration and no T_2, almost all patients with node metastases being T_3. There were, on average, 10.09 nodes per case (range 2–26 nodes). As previously stated, node involvement was discovered in 10 patients, an incidence of 19.23%. Perineal radical prostatectomy was performed on two patients during the same surgical procedure. A posterior histopathological study of paraffin-embedded sections revealed tumour infiltration in one patient, which finding should underline the importance of considering the presence of false negatives in preoperative studies. In general, no correspondence was found between the macroscopic aspect of the nodes and their histological nature.

Nodal dissection was performed unilaterally in seven cases for various reasons: in three patients, study of fresh-frozen specimens indicated tumour invasion and surgery was therefore abandoned; in the other four cases, this was done because of anatomical problems relating to the surgical field (impossibility of identification of anatomical structures in two cases and the presence of multiple peritoneal adhesions in the other two). In the latter four cases, no contralateral nodal involvement was found in open surgery.

The mean surgical time was 2.49 h (range 4–1.33 h). Progress along the learning curve has enabled surgical time to be reduced by 0.63 h. Comparing the first 25 cases with the subsequent 27, the average time has fallen from 2.8 to 2.16 h. Analysis of the authors' last 15 cases has shown an average surgical time of 1.8 h without substantial modification of the extent of the anatomical dissection.

Average hospital stay has been 2 days (range 1–7 days). There has been an (unquantified) reduction in the use of analgesics in the immediate postoperative period compared with open surgery.

The authors have statistically analysed the predictive value for node involvement of several factors in prostate cancer. Statistically significant evaluations have been performed relating ranges of PSA and positive nodes: the distribution of patients by PSA range has shown a significant increase for node involvement about 20 ng/ml. The same study applied to the Gleason score has shown a significant increase for node involvement with a score equal to or greater than 7.

With reference to the different cutoff points chosen for PSA and the Gleason score, either independently or in association, a Gleason score equal to 7 and PSA equal to 40 show greater accuracy in predicting the existence of node involvement (Table 9.1). Eight patients (80% of the cases with nodal invasion) presented a Gleason score equal to or greater than 7. The mean PSA value in the group of patients with negative (N–) nodes was 15.75 and in the group with positive (N+) nodes it was 52.74, the difference being statistically significant ($p=0.0001$). The mean Gleason score in the N– patients was 5.74 and in the N+ patients it was 7.2. ($p=0.0006$).

The overall rate of complications was 13.46% (7/52 patients), with no patient mortality. The most serious complications involved four cases (7.7%); these occurred intraoperatively in two cases and the other two in the postoperative period, all in the initial stages of the authors' experience (the first 19 patients). In the first group, the first case was of injury to the wall of the left external iliac artery due to accidental electrocoagulation in a diabetic patient with severe atheromatosis: the second patient suffered a bladder puncture while the area of the umbilical ligament was being dissected. An immediate laparotomy was performed on the first patient, with repair of the vascular injury with a prosthesis. The second case was quickly resolved with a laparoscopic endosuture, without stopping the operation. In the second group, the

Predictive value	Factor		
	Gleason 7*	PSA 40 ng/ml[†]	Gleason 7 + PSA > 40
Sensitive (%)	80	50	87.5
Specificity (%)	76.47	92.31	70.96
PPV[‡] (%)	50	57.14	43.75
NPV[§] (%)	92.86	90	95.65
Efficacy (%)	77.77	85.1	74.35

*Gleason score ≥ 7
[†]Prostate-specific antigen ≥ 40 ng/ml
[‡]PPV, positive predictive value.
[§]NPV, negative predictive value.

Table 9.1. Statistical evaluation of predictive value, for node involvement, of various factors in prostate cancer

first case was of an ischaemic ureteral fistula caused by excessive electrocoagulation of the surgical field; this was resolved with a temporary diversion using a percutaneous nephrostomy. The second patient had a haematoma of the anterior abdominus rectus muscle secondary to accidental vascular injury during the use of trocars.

Minor complications occurred in three patients (5.8%), comprising one case of paralytic ileus, one of penoscrotal emphysema (with a prior inguinal herniorrhaphy), and one of omental emphysema; all resolved spontaneously. There was no incidence of pulmonary thromboembolism, deep vein thrombosis, lymphocoele, hypercapnia, or pain of the shoulder secondary to irritation by the pneumoperitoneum.

Discussion

Development of laparoscopic technique has transformed lymphadenectomy into a genuine alternative to open surgery. Four years' experience of these techniques now enables the accumulated experience of various teams to be evaluated. An objective analysis of the technique should take into account such fundamental aspects such as its diagnostic reliability, its advantages and disadvantages in comparison to classical procedures, its complications and its current indications.

Parra[37] compared laparoscopic lymphadenectomy and open surgery lymphadenectomy in two groups of patients of similar ages and clinical stages; he obtained 10.7 and 11 nodes per case, respectively, showing a lack of significant differences between the two groups. Similar results were found by Griffith[38] with 31 patients: he obtained 11.3 nodes per case laparoscopically and 13.2 using conventional means. In his series, Schuessler[39] reported the high value of 45.3 nodes per case, which is difficult to reproduce. Schuessler insisted on the need to include nodal dissection of the iliac artery to avoid false negatives and low staging. In his series, he warns of the existence of up to 30% in cases with exclusive involvement of the external iliac group, corroborating the results of other classical series, such as those of Nicholson[40] (17%), Arduino[41] (57%) and Bruse[42] (54%).

The global percentage of cases with nodal involvement in the series of Schuessler,[39] Parra,[37] Kerbl,[43] Bowsher,[44] Rukstalis[45] and Griffith[38] was 23% (20/86), 25% (3/12), 30% (9/30), 16.7% (2/12), 21.4% (15/70) and 3% (1/31), respectively. Comparable results have been achieved by the present authors. Griffith attributes the low incidence in his series to the initial learning stages. In general, authors agree that the technique has a high degree of diagnostic reliability and that the volume of nodes detected is similar to that obtained with the conventional technique.

The laparoscopic procedure inherently has a series of advantages in that it is more comfortable for the patient and permits rapid postoperative recovery; it gives rise to less dependence on analgesics, a shorter stay in hospital (with consequent reduction of costs), a more rapid reintegration to the workplace and better aesthetic results.

The average hospital stay has been reported as 1, 1.2, 2, 1.7, 1.0 and 1.6 days,[37–39,43–45] which is much less than that following conventional open lymphadenectomy surgery.

In all the series an objective reduction in the average dose of analgesics and of postoperative haemorrhage is reported. Kerbl[43] compares various parameters in the two techniques; including average days of convalescence at home (4.94 vs 42.9 days), and the interval to normal resumption of work (10.8 vs 65.5 days). One of the less favourable aspects of the laparoscopic technique is the surgical time invested, which is much greater than with traditional surgery — 185, 184, 150, 199, 110 and 156 min.[37–39,43–45] However, these times will be reduced once the learning curve has been mastered by the different teams. It is still an expensive technique owing to the high cost of the instruments; these costs can be justified, however, by the short hospital stay, low morbidity and reduced convalescence.[46]

The technique is not exempt from morbidity.[47–49] Kavoussi[49] performed an important multicentre study reviewing the complications associated with this surgery with the collaboration of eight hospital centres as a reference, and included a total of 372 cases. The study reflects complications of 15% (56 patients) globally, 25% of which manifested themselves during surgery. In 13 cases (23%) open surgery was necessary to resolve the problem; in seven of these cases such surgery was performed immediately and in six cases the procedure was deferred. The most frequent type of complication was vascular (20%), occurring during trocar manipulation or nodal dissection (injury to the epigastric artery, umbilical ligament, obturator vein, external iliac artery superficial veins of the abdominal wall, haematoma of the anterior rectus abdominus muscle, and pelvic haematoma). The remaining complications in order of frequency were genitourinary problems (18%), visceral organ injury (14%), mechanical or paralytic ileus (12.7%), lower-limb deep vein thrombosis (9%), lymphoedema (9%), problems relating to anaesthesia (3.6%), and transitory paresis of the obturator nerve (3.6%).

No patient died as a result of surgery. In the opinion of Kavoussi et al.,[49] the initial results reflect a technique that is currently in a phase of expansion and learning. Parra[37] has mentioned a reduction in the genital and lower-limb lymphoedema that occurs so frequently in the wider dissection involved in conventional techniques. Griffith[38] noted a reduced incidence of paralytic ileus and thromboembolism, due to early resumption of ambulation by his patients. There is no doubt that correct selection of patients, correct selection of a surgical team (with prior training in laparoscopy), and improvements in surgical instruments will avoid numerous complications in the future; it is essential to make progress along the learning curve.

The indications for the laparoscopic technique are controversial and currently subject to discussion. Indications will be established when results provide a therapeutic standpoint and when the expected incidence of ganglion involvement of any specific patient justifies the procedure. There is a series of patients in whom lymphatic involvement is expected to be so low that systematic intervention would not be indicated. However, it is difficult to pinpoint such patients and to do so we state several considerations. At present the overall incidence of nodal invasion is not as high as that reported in the 1970s and 1980s; Table 9.2 shows 20–30% of positive nodes present in low stages (A and B).

A rapid review of the first series published[32,33] indicates that initially the indications were very broad, with few limitations, in all patients subject to radical surgery, even in very low stages; generally, other predictive factors (such as PSA and Gleason score) were not evaluated. Partin et al.,[56] on the other hand, noted that the combination of clinical staging, PSA and Gleason score permit an earlier prediction of the nodal situation; thus, these become prognostic factors defining the group of high-risk patients who will be the real beneficiaries of the laparoscopic technique.

What has occurred since 1990, and what results have been obtained? In the first place, the current series refer to a much lower node

Series	Ref. no.*	Year	No. of patients	Percentage of positive nodes at clinical stage			
				A_1	A_2	B_1	B_2
McLaughlin	50	1976	60	–	–	21	30
Paulson	51	1979	84	4	25	16	25
Grossman	52	1980	82	0	53	17	29
Hackler	53	1980	517	0	24	17	42
Flanigan	54	1985	53	–	0	0	42
Oesterling	55	1987	275	0	9	4	33
Gervasi	11	1989	511	–	22	21	37

* As in reference list

Table 9.2. Nodal involvement documented in previous series, according to clinical stage

involvement rate. In the last studies by Petros[57] and Danella[58] there was a decrease in the overall percentage of unsuspected nodal involvement in localized cancer of the prostate from 20 to 4.3% (before and after 1986) and from 20 to 5.7% (before and after 1988), respectively. This is explained in terms of an improvement in early detection techniques (PSA etc.) that allow earlier intervention in the natural history of prostate cancer.

It is evident, therefore, that an attempt should be made to differentiate patients with a low risk of node involvement from those at high risk, the latter group being where staging lymphadenectomy is really indicated. There is a group of patients in whom node involvement can be anticipated as being so low that the technique would not be routinely indicated.

There is universal agreement[37–39,43] that patients who are going to receive definitive radiotherapy or perineal prostatectomy should be treated with laparoscopy. However, Kerbl[43] does not practise this technique when the tumour presents the following three characteristics simultaneously: (1) clinical stage inferior to B_2 with PSA less than or equal to 20 ng/ml; (2) Gleason score less than 6; (3) no prior history of positive nodes.

Parra[37] performs the laparoscopic technique in patients with an elevated acid phosphates and normal bone scan and in cases where tumours are poorly differentiated and/or with an elevated PSA (without establishing figures).

Griffith[38] justifies the methodology if one of the following characteristics is met: (1) Gleason score greater than or equal to 8; (2) unfavourable histology (poorly differentiated); (3) elevated prostatic acid phosphatase; (4) seminal vesicle involvement (the present authors' group excludes these patients); or (5) clinical stage C.

Kerbl[43] advocates the technique when patients are candidates for retropubic prostatectomy, and present one or more of the following characteristics: (1) clinical stage of B_2, C, D_0 and/or a negative ganglion biopsy with a needle-directed CT; (2) PSA value greater than or equal to 40 ng/ml; (3) a Gleason score greater than or equal to 8.

According to Chodak[59] the technique is indicated at a T_{2b} or T_{2c} clinical stage, where the PSA is greater than 20 ng/ml, and the Gleason score is greater than 6.

Rukstalis[45] performs the technique in patients with localized cancer and a PSA value greater than 20 ng/ml or a Gleason score greater than or equal to 7, before radical surgery or radiotherapy.

Danella[58] concludes that routine laparoscopic nodal dissection is unnecessary in clinically localized prostatic cancer, except in patients with a PSA value greater than 40 ng/ml, or in those with a Gleason score greater than or equal to 7 together with a PSA value above 15 ng/ml.

The experience of the present authors' group over the last 4 years can be summarized as follows:

1. An initial phase, in which lymphadenectomy was indicated for all patients who were candidates for radical surgery of curative intent.
2. After analysis of the first results, a very small incidence of node involvement at low stages (T_1 and T_{2a}) was observed, which was contrary to historical opinion in this respect. The authors therefore started to restrict the procedure to patients with stages equal to or greater than T_{2b}, or those less than T_{2b} but with risk factors such as a PSA value above 20 and/or Gleason score greater than or equal to 7. It should be stressed that the authors' staging protocol included echographically directed biopsies of the seminal vesicles. Involvement of the seminal vesicles means disseminated disease, due to which patients are excluded from radical surgery.
3. Currently, in the light of the above, the present authors have a more restrictive policy, with the objective of performing lymphadenectomy in those groups of patients with a high probability of node involvement. The procedure is now indicated in patients with stage T_3, independent of PSA or Gleason score; for stages lower than T_3 the procedure is indicated only where there are associated risk factors (PSA equal to or greater than 20 and/or Gleason score equal to or greater than 7).

Once more experience has been gained and the results have been subjected to statistical analysis, the indications for laparoscopic lymphadenectomy can be optimized.

References

1. Parkin D M, Laara E, Muir C S. Estimate of the worldwide frequency of sixteen major cancers in 1980. Int J Cancer 1988; 41: 184–197
2. Teillac P, Bron J, Tobolski F et al. Dépistage du cancer de la prostate. Etude de 600 cas. Ann Urol 1990; 24: 37–41
3. Jewett H J. Prostatic cancer: a personal view of the problem. J Urol 1984; 131: 845–849
4. Goodman C M, Chisholm G D. Presentación y supervivencia en el adenocarcinoma de próstata. Análisis de 438 casos consecutivos estudiados a lo largo de 10 años. Arch Esp Urol 1989; 42(suppl.2): 117–123
5. Kozlowski J M, Grayhack J T. Carcinoma of the prostate. In: Gillenwater J Y, Grayhack J T, Howards S S, Duckett J W (eds) Adult and pediatric urology. Chicago: Year Book Medical, 1987; 2: 1126–1130

6. Gibbons R P, Correa R J, Brannen G E, Weisman R M. Total prostatectomy for clinically localized prostatic cancer: long term results. J Urol 1989; 144: 564–566

7. National Institutes of Health Consensus Conference. The management of clinically localized prostate cancer. J Urol 1987; 138: 1369–1375

8. Lepor H, Kimball A W, Walsh P C. Cause-specific actuarial survival analysis. A useful method for reporting data in men with clinically localized carcinoma of the prostate. J Urol 1989; 141: 82–84

9. Sack N H, Lane W W, Priore R L, Murphy G P. Prostate cancer. Treated at a categorical centre, 1980–1983. Urology 1986; 27: 205–213

10. Sanz Velez J I, Gil Sanz M J, Allepuz Losa C, Rioja Sanz L A. Cáncer de próstata: aspectos actuales del diagnóstico. Actas Urol Esp 1991; 15: 518–526

11. Gervasi L A, Mata J, Easley J D et al. Prognostic significance of lymph nodal metastases in prostate cancer. J Urol 1989; 142: 332–336

12. Jing B S, Wallace S, Zornoza J. Metastases to retroperitoneal and pelvic lymph nodes. Radiol Clin North Am 1982; 20: 511-529

13. Morgan C L, Calkins R F, Cavalcanti E J. Computed tomography in the evaluation, staging and therapy of carcinoma of the bladder and prostate. Radiology 1981; 140: 751–761

14. Teillac P, Leroy M, Rain J D et al. Premiers résultats chez l'homme de l'inmunolymphoscintigraphie dans le cancer de prostate. Ann Med Interne (Paris) 1989; 140: 20–24

15. Larson A, Arnberg H, Maripy E et al. Radioinmunodetection of prostatic cancer with I-labelled antibody against prostatic specific antigen. Scand J Urol Nephrol Suppl 1988; 110: 149–153

16. Weinerman P M, Arger P H, Coleman B G et al. Pelvic adenopathy from bladder cancer and prostate cancer detection by rapid sequence computed tomography. A J R 1983; 140: 95–99

17. Levine N S, Arger P H, Coleman B G et al. Detecting lymphatic metastases from prostatic carcinoma: superiority of C.T. A J R 1981; 137: 207

18. Giri P G, Walsh J W, Hazra T A et al. Role of computed tomography in the evaluation and management of carcinoma of the prostate. Int J Radiat Oncol Biol Phys 1982; 8: 283

19. Biondetti P R, Lee J K, Ling D, Catalona W J. Clinical stage B prostatic carcinoma: staging with MR imaging. Radiology 1987; 162: 325

20. Hricak H, Dooms G C, Jefrey R B et al. Prostatic carcinoma: staging by clinical assesment, C.T. and M.R. imaging. Radiology 1987; 162: 331

21. Mukamel E, Hannah J, Basrbaric Z et al. The value of computerized tomography scan and magnetic resonance imaging in staging prostatic carcinoma: comparison with the clinical and histological staging. J Urol 1986; 136: 1231–1233

22. Poon P Y, McCallum R W, Henkelman H M. Magnetic resonance imaging of the prostate. Radiology 1985; 154: 143–149

23. Donohue R E, Mani J H, Whitesel J A et al. Intraoperative and early complications of staging pelvic lymph node dissection in prostatic adenocarcinoma. Urology 1990; 35: 223–227

24. McDowel G C, Johnson J V, Tenney D M et al. Pelvic lymphadenectomy for staging clinically localized prostate cancer. Indications, complications and results in 217 cases. Urology 1990; 35: 476-482

25. Kramalowsky E W, Narayana A S, Platz C E et al. The frozen section in lymphadenectomy for carcinoma of the prostate. J Urol 1984; 131: 899

26. Epstein J I, Oesterling J E, Egleston J C et al. Frozen section detection of lymph node metastases in prostatic carcinoma: accuracy in grossly and uninvolved pelvic lymphadenectomy specimens. J Urol 1986; 136: 1234

27. Hermansen D K, Whitmore W F Jr. Frozen section lymph node analysis in pelvic lymphadenectomy for prostate cancer. J Urol 1988; 139: 1071–1074

28. Bartel M. Die Retroperitoneoskopie. Eine endosckopische Methode zur Inspektion und bioptischen. Untersuchung des retroperitonealen Raumes. Zbl Chir 1969; 94: 377

29. Hald T, Rasmussen F. Extraperitoneal pelvioscopy: a new aid in staging of lower urinary tract tumors. A preliminary report. J Urol 1988; 124: 245–248

30. Mazeman E, Wurtz A, Gilliot P, Biserte J. Extraperitoneal pelvioscopy in lymph node staging of bladder and prostatic cancer. J Urol 1992; 147: 366–370

31. Mazeman E, Lemaitre L, Wurtz A, Gilliot P. Exploration ganglionnaire dans les cancers de la prostate et de la vessie. Prog Urol 1991; 1: 321–332

32. Schuessler W W, Vancaillie T G, Reich H, Griffith D P. Transperitoneal endosurgical lymphadenectomy in patients with localized prostate cancer. J Urol 1991: 145: 988–991

33. Rioja Sanz C, Minguez Peman J M, Blas Marin M et al. Linfadenectomía laproscópia para estadiaje ganglionar en cáncer prostático: experiencia inicial. Actas Urol Esp 1991; 15: 515–517

34. Rioja Sanz C, Blas Marin M, Minguez Peman J M, Rioja Sanz L A. Linfadenectomía laparoscópica. Arch Esp Urol 1993; 46: 593–601

35. Harrison S H, Seale-Hawkins C, Schum C W et al. Correlation between side of palpable tumor and side of pelvic lymph node metastasis in clinically localized prostate cancer. Cancer 1992; 69: 750–754

36. Winfield H N, Schuessler W W. Pelvic lymphadenectomy: limited and extended. In: Laparoscopic Urology. St Louis: Quality Medical Publishing, 1992

37. Parra R O Andrus C, Boullier J. Staging laparoscopic pelvic lymph node dissection: comparison of results with open pelvic lymphadenectomy. J Urol 1992; 147: 875–878

38. Griffith D P, Schuessler W W, Nickell K G, Meaney J T. Laparoscopic pelvic lymphadenectomy for prostatic adenocarcinoma. Urol Clin North Am 1992; 19: 407–415

39. Schuessler W W, Pharand A, Vancaillie T G. Laparoscopic standard pelvic node dissection for carcinoma of the prostate: is it accurate? J Urol 1993; 150: 898–901

40. Nicholson T C, Richie J P. Pelvic lymphadenectomy for stage B1 adenocarcinoma of the prostate. J Urol 1977; 117: 199

41. Arduino L J, Glucksman M A. Lymph node metastases in early carcinoma of the prostate. J Urol 1962; 88: 91

42. Bruce A W, O'Cleireachain F, Morales A, Awad S A. Carcinoma of the prostate: a critical look at staging. J Urol 1977: 319

43. Kerbl K, Clayman R V, Petros J A et al. Staging pelvic lymphadenectomy for prostate cancer: a comparison of laparoscopic and open techniques J Urol 1993; 150: 396–399

44. Bowsher W G, Clarke A, Clarke D G, Costello A J. Laparoscopic pelvic lymph node dissection. Br J Urol 1992; 70: 276–279

45. Rukstalis D B, Gerber G S, Vogelzang N J et al. Laparoscopic pelvic lymph node dissection: a review of 103 consecutive cases. J Urol 1994; 151: 670–674

46. Troxel S, Winfield H N. Comparative financial analysis of laparoscopic versus open pelvic lymph node dissection for men with cancer of the prostate. J Urol 1994; 151: 675–680

47. Capelouto C C, Kavoussi L R. Complications of laparoscopic surgery. Urology 1993; 42: 2–12

48. Parra R O, Hagood P G, Boullier J A et al. Complications of laparoscopic urological surgery: experience at St Louis University. J Urol 1994; 151: 681–684

49. Kavoussi L R, Sosa E, Chandhoke P et al. Complications of laparoscopic pelvic lymph node dissection. J Urol 1993; 142: 322–325

50. McLaughlin A P, Saltzstein S L, McCullough D L, Gittes R F. Prostatic carcinoma: incidence and location of unsuspected lymphastic metastases. J Urol 1976; 115: 89

51. Paulson D F and Oro-Oncology Research Group. The impact of current staging procedures in assessing disease extent of prostatic adenocarcinoma. J Urol 1979; 121: 300

52. Grossman I C, Carpiniello V, Greenberg S H et al. Staging pelvic lymphadenectomy for carcinoma of the prostate: review of 91 cases. J Urol 1980; 124: 632

53. Hackler R H, Texter J H Jr. Evaluation and management of early stages of carcinoma of prostate. Urology 1980; 15: 329

54. Flanigan R C, Mohler J L, King C T et al. Preoperative lymph node evaluation in prostatic cancer patients who are surgical candidates: the role lymphangiography and computerized tomography scanning with directed fine needle aspiration. J Urol 1985; 134: 84

55. Oesterling J E, Brendler C B, Epstein J I et al. Correlation of clinical stage, serum prostatic acid phosphatase and preoperative Gleason grade with final pathological stage in 275 patients with clinically localized adenocarcinoma of the prostate. J Urol 1987; 138: 92

56. Patin A W, Yoo J, Carter H B et al. The use of prostate specific antigen, clinical stage and Gleason score to predict pathological stage in men with localized prostate cancer. J Urol 1993; 150: 110–114

57. Petros J A, Catalona W. Lower incidence of unsuspected lymph node metastases in 521 consecutive patients with clinically localized prostate cancer. J Urol 1992; 147: 1574–1575

58. Danella J F, déKernion J B, Smith R B, Steckel J. The contemporary incidence of lymph node metastases in prostate cancer: implications for laparoscopic lymph node dissection. J Urol 1993; 149: 1488–1491

59. Chodak G.W. The role of laparoscopic lymphadenectomy in the management of carcinoma of the prostate. Urol Int 1994; 1: 6

10

Is lymph node dissection still needed in radical prostatectomy?

P. Perrin   J. P. Fendler
M. Devonec

Introduction

The opportunity for lymph node dissection in radical prostatectomy is controversial. Lymphadenectomy can give essential prognostic information but has no therapeutic benefit.[1] Moreover, lymph node involvement now occurs less frequently because of better selection of patients before surgery.

The aim of this study was to assess the relationship between capsular status and lymph nodes, and to determine whether assessment of capsular penetration by biopsy could alter the decision to carry out lymph node dissection.

Patients and methods

The study included 209 cases of retropubic radical prostatectomy performed between 1986 and 1993 for prostate cancer of clinical stages T_1–T_2. Lymph node dissection was performed in each case. Prostatectomy specimens were studied according to McNeal's procedure.[2]

Capsular penetration was defined as tumour extension into the periprostatic soft tissue without involvement of seminal vesicles. Three groups of patients were defined according to capsular penetration criteria described by Epstein.[3–5] (1) established capsular penetration (ECP), (2) focal capsular penetration (FCP) and (3) no capsular penetration (NCP).

On the basis of capsular status, in each group nodal involvement and the rate of recurrence of nodes was studied, with a mean follow-up of 3.5 years. A detectable serum prostate-specific antigen (PSA) level (up to 0.3 ng/ml) was considered to indicate failure of treatment.

Results

Of the 209 patients, only 67 (32%) were in the NCP group; 142 patients (68%) had capsular penetration by tumour, comprising 33 FCP patients (16%) and 109 ECP patients (52%) (Table 10.1).

Of the 67 patients with intracapsular tumours, none had nodal involvement. In patients with FCP, only 5 (15%) had positive pelvic lymph nodes. Of patients with ECP, up to 31 (28%) had lymph node metastases.

Positive margins were found in 57% of ECP patients — 14/31 (45%) in N+ patients and 48/78 (61%) in N– patients. In FCP patients, positive margins occurred in 21% of cases (7/33). In this group, the positive margin rate was 20% in N+ patients (1/5) and 21% in N– patients (6/28). Of the NCP patients, 17/67 (25%) had surgically positive margins (Table 10.2).

Table 10.3 shows biological recurrence rates (rising PSA level) in radical prostatectomy patients according to capsular penetration and lymph node involvement. In patients with intact capsules (NCP), only 21% (14/67) showed biological progression of the disease, with a rising PSA level. In FCP patients, an increased PSA occurred in 32% (9/28) of patients with negative nodes and in 80% (4/5) of those with positive nodes. In patients in the ECP group, the overall progression rate was 73%, being 71% in N– patients and 74% in N+ patients. Moreover, in this group the positive margin rate was higher in N– patients than in N+ patients.

Discussion

Recent prostatectomy series have shown that lymph nodes were involved in only 5–10% of cases.[6,7]

Nodal involvement	Capsular penetration*		
	Establishment	Focal	None
N+	31 (28)	5 (15)	0 (0)
N–	78	28	67
Total	109 (52)	33 (16)	67 (32)

*No. of patients; percentage in parentheses.

Table 10.1. Relationship between capsular status and lymph node involvement in 209 radical prostatectomy specimens

Stage*	Positive margins	
	No. of patients	%
pT_2	17/67	25
pT_{3f}	7/33	21
pT_{3e}	62/109	57
Total	86/209	41

*pT_2 = patients with no capsular penetration; pT_{3f} = patients with focal capsular penetration; pT_{3e} = patients with established capsular penetration.

Table 10.2. The positive margin rate according to pathological stage and capsular status

Lymph node involvement	Capsular penetration[†]		
	Established	Focal	None
N+	22/31 (71)	4/5 (80)	0
N–	58/78 (74)	9/28 (32)	14/67 (21)
Total	80/109 (73)	13/33 (39)	14/67 (21)

*Mean follow-up 3.5 years; [†]no. of patients; percentages in parentheses

Table 10.3. Biological recurrence rate* (rising PSA level) according to capsular status and lymph node involvement in 209 patients undergoig radical prostatectomy.

Assessment of preoperative capsular status may have an important bearing on therapy and prognosis. Patients with no capsular extension are excellent candidates for radical prostectomy: their pelvic nodes are not involved by tumour and lymph node dissection is unnecessary. In such cases, the morbidity of lymph node dissection[8] may be greater than its benefit.

In theory, patients in the ECP group are good candidates for radical surgery, because of the high rate of positive margins (57%). Moreover, about one-third of such patients will have positive nodes. Surprisingly, in this group, N– and N+ patients present with an identical prognosis, in terms of biological progression. Nodes are not the major prognostic factor in these cases. Lymph node dissection may be of interest for staging but is not useful for assessment of prognosis.

Patients in the FCP group are potential candidates for radical prostectomy. Epstein[5] showed that focal capsular penetration by tumour was of low prognostic significance in itself. Nevertheless, 16% of these patients present with nodal involvement, which significantly modifies prognosis (80% vs 32% biological progression). In this group, prognosis is not dependent on capsular status but is related to node status. In such cases, lymph node dissection may have a diagnostic and prognostic interest. Unfortunately, only a few cases (33/209, 16% in the study reported here) are concerned.

There are no precise parameters or indices for prediction of capsular status. Rectal examination can discriminate T_3 tumours from T_2 tumours in only 45% of cases. The ability of magnetic resonance imaging to assess capsular penetration is disappointing.[9] Use of the preoperative serum PSA level and tumour grade to predict established capsular penetration, which has been suggested by Partin,[10] seems to be difficult to apply on an individual basis.

Only biopsies can give direct optimal information on capsular status before radical treatment. Improvement of the biopsy technique, with better capsular assessment, is necessary for accurate staging of prostate cancer to facilitate the decision on whether to perform lymph node dissection during radical prostatectomy.

Conclusions

The decision to carry out lymph node dissection in radical prostatectomy should be related to assessment of prostatic capsular status. In pT_2 tumours, lymphadenectomy may not be necessary because of the extremely low rate of lymph node involvement.

In pT_3 tumours with established capsular penetration, one-third have positive nodes. Moreover, in such cases the progression rate does not appear to depend on node status: biological failure occurs in the same proportions whether the nodes are involved or not.

Lymph node dissection may be of most interest in cases of pT_3 tumours with focal capsular penetration. In such cases, lymph node status could strongly affect the prognosis. The information gleaned from lymph node dissection may be vital in these patients.

Improvement of the biopsy technique with accurate assessment of capsular status must be achieved before radical prostatectomy is performed.

References

1. Cheng C W, Bergtralh E J, Zincke J L. Stage D1 prostate cancer. A non randomized comparison of conservative treatment options versus radical prostatectomy. Cancer 1993; 71 (suppl 3) 996–1004
2. McNeal J E, Bostwick D G, Kindrachuk R A et al. Patterns of progression in prostate cancer. Lancet 1986; 1: 60–63
3. Epstein J I. Evaluation of radical prostatectomy capsular margins of resection. Am J Surg Pathol 1990; 14: 626–632
4. Epstein J I, Pizov G, Walsh P C. Correlation of pathologic findings with progression following radical prostatectomy. Cancer 1993; 71: 3582–3593.
5. Epstein J I, Carmichael M J, Pizov V G, Walsh P C. Influence of capsular penetration following radical prostatectomy: a study of 196 cases with long term follow-up. J Urol 1993; 150: 135–141.
6. Danella J F, deKernion J B, Smith R B, Steckel J. The contemporary incidence of lymph node metastasis in prostate cancer: implications for laparoscopic lymph node dissection. J Urol 1993; 149: 1488–1491
7. Bundrick W S, Culkin D J, Mata J A et al. Evaluation of the current incidence of nodal metastasis from prostate cancer. J Surg Oncol 1993; 52: 269–271
8. Donohue R E, Mani J H, Whitesel J A et al. Intraoperative and early complications of staging pelvic node dissection in prostatic adenocarcinoma. Urology 1990; 35: 223–227
9. Outwater E K, Gomella L G, Peterson R. Assessment of diagnostic criteria for capsular penetration on endorectal MR images of the prostate. J Urol 1994; 151: 506A (abstr 1114)
10. Partin A W, Yoo J, Carter H B et al. The use of prostate specific antigen, clinical stage and Gleason score to predict pathological stage in men with localized prostate cancer. J Urol 1993; 150: 110–115

Frozen section in pelvic lymphadenectomy for staging of adenocarcinoma of the prostate

11

R. E. Donohue

Introduction

The year 1993 marks the one-hundredth anniversary of the introduction of the frozen section into medicine in the United States. Cullen returned from Germany to Johns Hopkins with Orth's solution, formaldehyde and frozen section was begun in the United States in 1893.[1]

Methods

A total of 230 consecutive patients who underwent staging pelvic lymphadenectomy using the modified dissection technique at the Denver VA Medical Center, Colorado, USA, underwent assessment of the dissected nodes by frozen section. The nodes in the specimen were identified and serially sectioned horizontally and vertically. Suspicious areas were selected for study. If all nodes appeared to be without disease, representative nodes were selected and studied. All nodal tissue was then fixed and evaluated using standard techniques.

Results

Twenty-five patients were identified by frozen section as having metastatic disease to their lymph nodes. This diagnosis was confirmed later by study of permanent sections of these nodes. Two hundred men were identified as having nodes free from disease at frozen section and later at review of the permanent section (Table 11.1).

One patient had suspicious nodes at frozen section but permanent section revealed a granulomatous reaction in the nodes. (Another

Frozen	Permanent Section	
section	Positive	Negative
Positive	25	1
Negative	4	200

Table 11.1. Assessment, by frozen and permanent section, of pelvic lymph nodes of 230 patients undergoing staging pelvic lymphadectomy at the Denver VA Medical Center, Colorado

patient had sarcoid identified at frozen section, confirmed at permanent section.)

Four patients had disease in the pelvic nodes undetected at frozen section. Two had disease in the afferent lymphatics to the node; one had disease in a node not sampled and one had obvious metastatic disease, missed by the pathologist.

Discussion

In 1891 Halsted, Professor of Surgery at Johns Hopkins University requested a frozen section on breast tissue from Welch,[1] Professor of Pathology. The operation was completed before the frozen section assessment. Two years later, using Orth's technique from Berlin, Cullen, a gynaecological pathology resident at Johns Hopkins, introduced the technique of frozen section to the United States. De Reimer suggested freezing tissue to harden it (1821). Wright suggested boiling the tissue in formalin.[1] Wilson froze the tissue and used a razor to cut the specimen and a microtome to cut the sections. Shultz-Brauns used compressed CO_2 and a microtome cooled to $-5°C$.

The literature on frozen section evaluation of the pelvic nodes dates from the late 1960s. Scott from Baylor was one of the first to suggest frozen section of the dissected lymph nodes and simultaneous radical prostatectomy.[2]

Prior to 1981, the dissection at pelvic lymphadenectomy included the obturator, hypogastric, external iliac and lower common iliac nodes. With the report of Fisher and Whitmore in 1981, the modified dissection, of the obturator and hypogastric nodes only, became popular.[3]

The largest series in the literature of positive nodes at frozen section are listed in Table 11.2. The incidence of positive nodes at frozen section from current series Epstein and Denver, was 10%, 54 of 540 patients.

Table 11.3 shows the incidence of false negatives at frozen section. In this situation, the frozen section report was negative for metastatic disease

Year	Series	Ref. no.	No. of patients	Positive nodes	
				No.	%
1971	Scott	2	82	?	–
1982	Catalona	4	75	16	21
	Fowler	5	40	5	12
1983	Sadlowski	6	42	10	24
1984	Kramolowsky	7	100	43	43*
1986	Epstein	8	310	29	9
1992	Walsh	9	234	6	3†
1994	Denver‡		230	25	9

*Only selected cases were reported.
†Nodes were cut but not frozen if they appeared negative.
‡Series reported here.

Table 11.2. Positive nodes at frozen section in major series

Series*	No. of patients	False-negative nodes	
		No.	%
Scott	82	3	3
Catalona	75	11	15
Fowler	40	3	8
Sadlowski	42	3	7
Kramolowsky	100	16	16
Epstein	310	11	4
Walsh	234	19	8
Denver	230	4	2

*Date, and ref no; as in Table 11.2.

Table 11.3. False-negative nodes at frozen section in major series

but the permanent sections returned positive. The incidence of false negative reports from Epstein and Denver was 2.7%, 15 of 540 reports.

The current incidence of positive nodes is shown in Table 11.4. The incidence of positive nodes, stage D_1, from the four most recent series, Epstein, Walsh, Catalona and Denver, is 10%, 129 of 1292 patients. Catalona reported that the incidence of positive nodes has fallen in the last few years in his series. The Denver experience supports his comment: with minimal numbers of stage C patients clinically undergoing standard

Series	Ref. no.	No. of patients	Positive nodes No.	Positive nodes %
Scott	2	82	?	?
Catalona	4	75	27	36
Fowler	5	40	8	20
Sadlowski	6	42	13	31
Kramolowsky	7	100	58	58
Epstein	8	310	40	13
Walsh	9	234	25	11
Catalona	10	518	35	7
Denver*		230	29	13

*Series reported here.

Table 11.4. Incidence of positive nodes at lymphadenectomy in major series

pelvic lymphadenectomy, the incidence of positive nodes with the dissection was 23%; the current modified dissection has a positive incidence of 13%.

Conclusions

The frozen section technique, celebrating its one-hundredth year in the United States, is an accurate and reliable method of node assessment for malignant disease. Its use in staging pelvic lymphadenectomy for localized prostatic carcinoma at the time of radical prostatectomy yields almost uniformly excellent results in the current series. Like surgery and the surgeon, the more often the surgical pathologist is called upon to exercise his skill in assessing nodes, the more proficient he becomes.

References

1. Wright J R. The development of the frozen section technique, the evolution of surgical biopsy and the origin of surgical pathology. Bull Hist Med 1985; 59: 295
2. Kopecky J, Laskowski M, Scott R. Radical retropubic prostatectomy in the treatment of prostatic carcinoma. J Urol 1971; 103: 641
3. Fisher H, Whitmore W F. The modified pelvic node dissection. AUA Abstr 1981; 299
4. Catalona W J, Stein A J. Accuracy of frozen section detection of lymph node metastases in prostatic cancer. J Urol 1982; 126: 460
5. Fowler J E, Torgerson L, McCloud D G, Stutzman R. Radical prostatectomy with pelvic lymph node dissection: observations on the accuracy of staging with lymph node frozen section. J Urol 1981; 126: 618

6. Sadlowski R W, Donahue R J, Richman A V *et al.* Accuracy of frozen section diagnosis in pelvic lymph node staging biopsies for adenocarcinoma of the prostate. J Urol 1983; 129: 324

7. Kramolowsky E V, Narayan A S, Platz C E, Leoning S. The frozen section in lymphadenectomy for carcinoma of the prostate. J Urol 1984; 131: 899

8. Epstein J I, Oesterling J E, Eggleston J C, Walsh P C. Frozen section detection of lymph node metastases in prostatic carcinoma: accuracy in grossly uninvolved pelvic nodes. J Urol 1986; 136: 1234

9. Burnett A L, Chan D W, Brendler C B, Walsh P C. The value of serum enzymatic acid phosphatase in the staging of localized prostate cancer. J Urol 1992; 148: 1832

10. Petros J A, Catalona W J. Lower incidence of unsuspected lymph node metastases in 521 consecutive patients with clinically localized prostate cancer. J Urol 1992; 147: 1574

Penis

Carcinoma of the penis

12

L. M. Harewood

Introduction

Carcinoma of the penis is one of only two urological malignancies for which lymph node surgery may be a curative, rather than a staging or palliative measure, the other being carcinoma of the testis. Hence, lymph node surgery for carcinoma of the penis is important and does make a difference in node-positive patients. Nevertheless, there remain many undecided issues, including the following:

1. Whether node surgery should be used, in patients with clinically negative nodes, as early systematic (adjunctive) or delayed therapeutic;
2. The place of pelvic lymph node surgery;
3. The relevance of the grade of tumour to surgery;
4. The type of surgery to be offered;
5. The type of incision to be used;
6. The role of radiotherapy to positive nodes.

This chapter is a review of recent literature, to address these issues.

Staging

Until very recently the commonest staging system was the Jackson system.[1] (Table 12.1) Jackson was a radiotherapist, and the system was used as a retrospective classification of patients, based on the findings at surgery, or the subsequent outcome of the patient. The system therefore

Stage	Penile cancer
I	Tumour confined to glans or prepuce.
II	Tumour extending onto shaft of penis.
III	Inguinal metastases that are operable.
IV	Involving adjacent structures; inoperable inguinal nodes; distant metastases.

Table 12.1. Jackson classification of penile cancer, 1966

is both pathological and retrospective, and hence is of limited clinical use. It has made interpretation of many papers published in recent years very difficult, as patients who are found to have operable inguinal metastases are automatically classified as stage III regardless of the presenting clinical state.

The TNM system of 1974 ref. 2 (Table 12.2) is a significant improvement as it is a prospective clinical classification, and hence is of prognostic value, and allows comparison of different series. Nevertheless, the classification of the primary lesion by size and invasion was found not to be the most relevant characteristic.

The TNM system of 1988 (ref. 3) (Table 12.3) is the most useful system as it classifies the primary lesion according to whether the corpora

Tumour	Nodes	Metastases
T_{is}: carcinoma in situ	N_0: no palpable nodes	M_0: no distant mets
T_1: <2cm superficial	N_1: movable unilateral nodes	M_1: distant metastases
T_2: >2cm minimal invasion	N_2: movable bilateral nodes	
T_3: >5cm or deep invasion	N_3: fixed nodes	
T_4: invading adjacent structures		

Table 12.2. TNM *staging of penile cancer, 1974*

Tumour	Nodes	Metastases
T_{is}: carcinoma in situ	N_0: No regional nodes	M_0: no distant metastases
T_1: invades subepithelial connective tissue	N_1: single superficial node	M_1: distant metastases
T_2: invades corpus spongiosum or cavernosum	N_2: multiple or bilateral nodes	
T_3: invades urethra or prostate	N_3: deep inguinal or pelvic nodes	
T_4: invades adjacent structures.		

Table 12.3. TNM *staging of penile cancer, 1988*

are invaded or not, which correlates best with the presence or absence of inguinal node metastases. Similarly, the most relevant nodal state is whether a single node or multiple nodes are involved. It should be the classification of choice in all future publications.

Incidence (Table 12.4)

Carcinoma of the penis is a rare disease in Western nations. In the USA its rate is 0.9/100 000 men, and in Australia its rate is 0.7/100 000 men, comparing with a rate for carcinoma of the prostate of 75/100 000 and 50/100 000 men, respectively. In Israel its rate is 0.1/100 000 men, presumably reflecting the rate of circumcision in that country.

Region	Country	Incidence	Reference
Western nations	USA	0.4% male malignancies 0.9/100 000 men/year	Persky (1977)[4]
	Australia	0.7/100 000 men/year	ACC Vic(1994)[5]
	France	1.14% male cancers	Bouchot (1989)[6]
	Canada	0.7/100 000 men/year	Persky (1977)[4]
	England	1.2/100 000 men/year	Persky (1977)[4]
	Scandinavian	1.3/100 000 men/year	Persky (1977)[4]
	Italy	0.5/100 000 men/year	Persky (1977)[4]
	Israel	0.1/100 000 men/year	Persky (1977)[4]
Asian nations	India	2% all malignancies (? 4% male) 1.6/100 000 yr	Kuruvilla (1971)[7] Ravi (1993)[8]
	Vietnam	11.5% male malignancies	Persky (1977)[4]
	Thailand	6.6% male malignancies	Persky (1977)[4]
	China	12% to 22% all cancers	Persky (1977)[4]
African nations	Uganda	12% male cancers 2.2/100 000 men/year	Persky (1977)[4]
	S. Africa	4.6/100 000 men/year Natal 1.7% Bantu male cancers	Persky (1977)[4]
	Kenya	1.9% male cancers	Persky (1977)[4]
	Nigeria	0.2/100 000 men/year	Persky (1977)[4]
S. American Nations	Brazil	2.1% all malignancies; up to 17% all malignancies some regions	Ornellas (1994)[9]
	Mexico	10% male cancers	Persky (1977)[4]
	Puerto Rico	20% males cancers 5/100 000 men/year	Persky (1977)[4]
	Columbia	2.3/100 000 men/year	Persky (1977)[4]
	Paraguay	8.6% all malignancies	Riveros (1962)[10]

Table 12.4. Geographic incidence of carcinoma of the penis

In other nations, however, the rate may be very high, and carcinoma of the penis may be the most common male urological malignancy. Thus it is not an uncommon malignancy and its impact on the health services in some countries is very high indeed. As such, it is an important cancer, and high-calibre data on its natural history and management is of the highest priority.

Can we predict the likelihood of lymph node metastases from the clinical presentation, stage and grade of the tumour?

Palpable inguinal lymph nodes are common at the time of presentation in from 28 to 64% of patients (Table 12.5). Nevertheless only 47–86% of patients with palpable inguinal nodes do in fact have histologically positive nodes, as found in patients undergoing systematic lymph node dissection (Table 12.6). Unilateral palpable nodes are more likely to be positive than bilateral palpable nodes, which is consistent with the fact that enlarged nodes may be reactive hyperplasia attributable to infection of the primary tumour. Fixed nodes, however, are always due to metastases. Patients with impalpable nodes may still have nodal metastases with an incidence ranging from 12 to 42%.

The best guide to the likelihood of inguinal metastases is the clinical stage. Patients with a superficially invasive tumour (stage T_1) or a tumour confined to the glans penis (stage 1) have a mean incidence of only 9% (range 4–42%) (Table 12.7). Patients with a tumour that is invading the corpora (T_2–T_4), or extending onto the shaft of the penis (stage II) have a mean incidence of 47% (range 21–66%). Hence it is these patients who are candidates for systematic node dissection.

Reference	No. of patients	Incidence of nodes*		
		Stage I, T_a, T_1	Stage II, T_2–T_4	Overall
Solsona (1992)[11]	66			22/66 (33)
Horenblas (1991)[12]	114			48/114 (42)
Bouchot (1989)[6]	40	T_1 1/9 (11)	T_{2-4} 19/31 (61)	20/40 (50)
Srinivas (1987)[13]	119			76/119 (64)
Narayana (1982)[14]	213			60/213 (28)
Nelson (1982)[15]	115			40/115 (35)

*Percentage in parentheses

Table 12.5. Incidence of nodes palpable at presentation

Reference	No. of patients	Incidence of positive nodes*				
		Stage N_0, impalpable nodes	Stage N_1, unilateral palpable	Stage N_2, bilateral palpable	Stage N_3, fixed nodes	Overall N+ palpable
Ornellas (1994)[9]	133	9/23 (39)	16/23 (70)	29/69 (42)	18/18 (100)	63/110 (57)
Solsona (1992)[11]	33	3/11 (27)			8/8 (100)	14/22 (64)
Young (1991)[16]	12	5/12 (42)				
Horenblas (1991)[12]	102	7/56 (12)				33/46 (72)
Bouchot (1989)[6]						11/15 (73)
Srinivas (1987)[13]		7/38 (18)				66/76 (87)
Fraley (1985)[17]	12	2/6 (33)	3/5 (60)	1/1 (100)		6/12 (50)
Nelson (1982)[15]	40					19/40 (47)

*Percentages in parentheses

Table 12.6. Incidence of histological positive nodes related to N stage: patients undergoing systematic LND

Reference	No. of patients	Incidence of positive nodes*		
		Stage I or T_1	Stage II or T_2–T_4	Stage III or T_3
Solsona (1992)[11]	66	T_1 1/24 (4)	T_{2-3} 27/42 (64)	$p = 0.001$
Young (1991)[16]	12	St I 5/12 (42)		
Pettaway (1991)[18]	53	T_1 1/16 (6)	T_2 15/37 (40)	
Fraley (1989)[19]	33	St I 0/15 (0)	St II 9/18 (50)	
McDougal (1986)[20]	28	St I 0/19 (0)	St II 6/9 (67)	
Fraley (1985)[17]	12		T_{2-4} 5/12 (42)	
Narayana (1982)[14]	177	St I 13/129 (10)	St II 5/24 (21)	St III 22/24 (92)
Mean	357	20/215 (9)	67/142 (47)	

*Percentages in parentheses

Table 12.7. Incidence of positive nodes related to tumour (T) stage

The grade of tumour is also important (Table 12.8). The mean incidence of nodal metastases in patients with well-differentiated tumours is only 14%; with moderately differentiated tumours the incidence is 72% and with poorly differentiated tumours 96%. The main change occurs as soon as the tumour is anything but well differentiated, with the incidence of moderate and poorly differentiated tumours

Reference	No. of patients	Well differentiated	Moderately differentiated	Poorly differentiated
Solsona (1992)[11]	66 All stages	7/36 (19)	15/23 (65)	6/7 (85)
	Stage T_1	0/19 (0)	1/4 (25)	0/1 (0)
	Stage T_{2-3}	7/17 (41)	14/19 (73)	6/6 (100)
Fraley (1989)[19]	54	1/19 (5)	15/19 (79)	16/16 (100)
Mean	120	8/55 (14)	30/42 (71)	22/23 (96)
			Combined	mod and poor 52/65 (80)

Percentages in parentheses.

Table 12.8. Incidence of positive nodes (both early and late) related to grade

combined being 80%. When both stage and grade are combined, it is clear that both are important, as patients with stage T_1 tumours are rarely anything but well differentiated, and rarely have metastases (Table 12.9). As soon as patients have more than a stage T_1 tumour the incidence of nodal metastases rises to 41% for well-differentiated tumours, up to 100% for poorly differentiated.

Reference	Stage	Incidence of positive nodes*		
		Well differentiated	Moderately differentiated	Poorly differentiated
Solsona (1992)[11]	T_1	0/19 (0)	1/4 (25)	0/1 (0)
	T_2-T_3	7/17 (41)	14/19 (74)	6/6 (100)

*Percentages in parentheses

Table 12.9. Incidence of positive nodes related to both stage and grade

What are the results of early systemic lymph node dissection (LND), and how do they compare with delayed therapeutic lymph node dissection?

The 5-year survival of patients undergoing immediate systematic LND is very good, ranging from 62 to 100%, depending on the stage of the tumour, with very little difference between stage T_1 and T_{2-4} tumours (Table 12.10). However, this may entail the generation of morbidity or even mortality from the node dissection itself, which may be significant. In patients with T_1 tumours the incidence of node metastases is only 9% (Table 12.7); hence a large number of patients may undergo an unnecessary procedure. The results of penile surgery only, with delayed LND if the patient develops clinically palpable or suspicious nodes, in patients with T_1 or stage I tumours is excellent, with a 65–100% 5-year survival. Patients with T_3 or stage II tumours, however, did poorly, with only a 15–36% survival. Hence the results of early compared with delayed LND depend very much on the stage of the tumour.

What is of very much more concern, however, is what happened to the patients with a T_{2-4} or stage II tumour, who had penile surgery only and had the nodes followed. Very few actually underwent node dissection (Table 12.11). Only 7–12% of patients with a stage II tumour received a

| Reference | Stage | Total no. of patients | 5-year survival* | | p value |
			Immediate systematic LND	Penile surgery only; delayed LND if suspicious	
Ornellas (1994)[9]	All	326	(62) n=102	(38) n=224	0.175 n.s.
Young (1991)[16]	I (T_1/T_2N_0)	26	(75) n=12	(77) n=14	n.s.
Fraley (1989)[19]	Stage I	15	4/4 (100)	10/11 (91) no LND	
	Stage II/III	38	15/18 (83)	3/20 (15)	
McDougal (1986)[20]	Stage I	19		19/19 (100)	
	Stage II	23	8/9 (89)	5/14 (36)	
Fraley (1985)[17]	$T_{1-2}N_0$	61	5/6 (83)	36/55 (65)	
	$T_{3-4}N_0$	12	7/7 (100)	1/5 (20)	
	T_{1-4} N+ (Stage III)	6	4/6 (67)	1/4 (25)	
Narayana (1982)[14]	Stage 1	129		5/129 died Ca penis. 96% survival	
	Stage III	24	12/24 died Ca penis (50)		

*Percentages in parentheses.

Table 12.10. Five-year survival systematic (adjunctive) LND versus penile surgery only with delayed LND if suspicious nodes develop: overall figures

Reference	No. of patients	T stage	Delayed LND*
Ornellas (1994)[9]	224	All	42/224 (19) 50 died Ca penis 8% 5 yr survival
Bouchot (1989)[6]	18	All	2/18 (11)
McDougal (1986)[20]	Total 33	Stage I	0/19 (0) No deaths from Ca
		Stage II	1/14 (7) Only 38% 5 yr survival
Fraley (1985)[19]	55	St I T1–2N0	6/54 (11); 11/54 (20) died Ca penis
	9	T2–4 (St II–III)	0/9 0%; 7/9 (78) died Ca penis
Narayana (1982)[14]	153	Stage I	15/129 (12); 15/129 died Ca
		Stage II	3/25 (12); 5/24 (21) died Ca penis

*Percentages in parentheses.

Table 12.11. Incidence of patients with initial penile surgery only progressing on to delayed inguinal lymphadenectomy for suspicious nodes

node dissection, but up to 78% of them died of carcinoma of the penis. This suggests very strongly that patients were either lost to follow-up, became inoperable under observation, or became metastatic during the delay.

Further information comes from investigating the outcome in patients undergoing LND who had positive nodes (Table 12.12). Patients undergoing immediate systematic LND who had positive nodes did well, with a 75–100% 5-year survival. If the patient had palpable nodes and underwent an immediate therapeutic LND, the results were still good, with up to 66% surviving 5 years. If, however, the LND was delayed until the nodes became suspect, the survival was abysmal, the best being 17%. The patients undergoing early systematic node dissection who are found to have positive nodes are those that would go on to require LND for subsequent nodal metastases. The survival of these patients is better with

Reference	Total no. of patients	Immediate systematic LND with positive nodes	Immediate therapeutic LND for positive nodes	Delayed therapeutic LND for positive nodes
Ornellas (1994)[9]	84	All stages: (29) n=47		(0) n=37
Young (1991)[16]	17	Stage I/II: 0/5 (0) n=5	Stage III: 0/7 (0)	0/5 (0) n=5
Fraley (1989)[19]	20	Stage III: 6/8 (75) T_2–T_4		1/12 (8)
McDougal (1986)[20]	22	Stage II: 5/6 (83)	Stage III: 10/15 (67)	0/1 (0)
Fraley (1985)[17]	12	$T_{2-3}N_0$: 2/2 (100)	T_{1-3} N_{1-2}: 2/4 (50)	1/6 (17)
Johnson (1984)[21]	22		T_{1-3}: (57) n=14	(13) n=8
Nelson (1982)[15]	17		Stage III: 2/17 (12)	
Johnson (1973)[22]	30			3/30(10)

*Percentages in parentheses

Table 12.12. Five-year survival: immediate systematic LND, immediate therapeutic LND and delayed therapeutic LND in patients with positive nodes

early rather than late LND, and makes a clear case for early surgery in patients who may have involved nodes. These figures also make it clear that node surgery in patients with involved nodes may be curative with no further treatment.

From the above discussion it seems clear that, for stage T_1 with impalpable nodes, penile surgery only, with close observation only, is the best management. Very few of these patients are likely to require later LND. Patients with T_1N+ (palpable nodes on clinical presentation) may be left for 6 weeks to see if the nodes disappear, with LND if the nodes persist. Unilateral nodes are more likely to be metastatic, and an immediate LND in conjunction with the penile surgery may be both justified and expeditious. Patients with higher-stage tumours, i.e. T_2 to T_4, should undergo immediate systematic LND dissection regardless of whether the nodes are palpable.

How does nodal involvement affect survival?

The presence of positive nodes is a poor prognostic indicator (Table 12.13), regardless of whether early surgery is undertaken. The extent of nodal involvement is also important (Table 12.14): when the deep inguinal

Reference	Stage	Five-year survival*		
		No. of patients	Nodes negative	Nodes positive
Ornellas (1994)[9]	All	102	(87)	(29)
Young (1991)[16]	I/II	12	5/7 (71)	0/5 (0)
Fraley (1989)[19]	II/III	18	9/9 (100)	6/9 (67)
McDougal (1986)[20]	II	9	3/3 (100)	5/6 (83)
Fraley (1985)[17]	T_{2-4}	6	4/4 (100)	2/3 (67)

*Percentage in parentheses.

Table 12.13. Five-year survival related to positive or negative nodes for patients undergoing systematic LND

Reference	No. of patients	Five-year survival*			
		Overall N+ve	N_1, N_2 superficial nodes +ve	N_3 Deep inguinal nodes +ve	Iliac nodes +ve
Srinivas (1987)[13]	78	22/78 (28)	14/22 (64)	8/56 (14)	0/11 (0)

*Percentage in parentheses.

Table 12.14. Five-year suvival related to extent of nodal disease

nodes are affected, the survival is poor; when the pelvic nodes are involved, the result is uniformly fatal.

When are the pelvic nodes involved?

Fortunately, pelvic node involvement is uncommon (Table 12.15) and occurs only in high-stage tumours, in conjunction with deep inguinal node involvement. When the pelvic nodes are affected, treatment should only be palliative, as the patient is incurable by any modality at that stage. Dissection of the pelvic nodes is indicated only in high-stage tumours where the deep inguinal nodes are positive, and then as a staging procedure only. Assimos and Jarow[24] have described laparoscopic pelvic lymph node dissection as a means of assessing the pelvic nodes in patients with carcinoma of the penis; this may have a place in these patients.

Reference	No. of patients	Stage	Incidence of positive nodes*	
			Inguinal	Iliac
Ornellas (1994)[9]	18	All		(0)
Catalona (1988)[23]	5	II, III	2/5 (40)	0/5 (0)
Srinivas (1987)[13]	79	All	54/79 (68)	11/79 (14)
		I/II N_0 (impalp)	0/25 (0)	0
		III N+	54/54 (100)	11/54 (20)
		N_1–N_2 superficial		1/42 (2.4)
		N_3 deep nodes		10/37 (27)
Johnson (1984)[21]	4	$T_{2–4}N_{1–2}$	4/4 (100)	0/4 (0)

*Percentages in parentheses.

Table 12.15. Incidence of positive pelvic (iliac) nodes

How does grade of tumour affect survival?

The grade of tumour is significant (Table 12.16). Fortunately, the majority of patients have well-differentiated tumours, which do quite well. Poorly differentiated tumours have a uniformly poor prognosis. These factors should also be taken into consideration in the management of patients with carcinoma of the penis.

Reference	Total no. of patients	Five-year survival*		
		Well differentiated, G_1	Moderately differentiated, G_2, G_3	Poorly differentiated, G_4
Ornellas (1994)[9]	327	(62) n=216	(57) n=95	(30) n=16
Maiche (1991)[25]	239	(82) n=120	(56) n=107	(28) n=12
Fraley (1989)[19]	54	18/19 (95)	9/19 (47)	3/16 (19)
Fraley (1985)[17]	37	19/20 (95)	8/13 (62)	1/4 (25)

*Percentages in parentheses.

Table 12.16. Five-year survival relating to grade of tumour

Reference	Type of dissection	No. of dissections	No. of patients	Mortality (%)	Necrosis (%)	Infection (%)	Lymphocoele (%)	Lymphoedema (%)
Ravi (1993)[8]	Inguinal	231			61: 17 severe	18	5	25; 4 severe
	Ilioinguinal	144		1.3 overall	78: 15 severe	17	11	30; 15 severe
	Ilioinguinal + reconstruction	30			0	0	0	27; 10 severe
Ornellas (1991)[26]	Bi-iliac	21	21	0	82: (5/21 severe)	0	0	9
	S-shaped	94	47	0	72; (30/47 severe)	0	4	32
	Gibson	85	44	0	5 (4/44) (1/44 severe)	15	9	16
Fraley (1989)[19]	Immediate double transverse		22		(1/22 minor; 3/22 severe)	(1/22 abscess)		
	Delayed double transverse		12		(2/12 minor; 5/12 severe)			
Catalona (1988)[23]	Modified	10	5	0	(1/5) 20	(1/5)20	(1/5) 20	(4/5) 80 min
McDougal (1986)[20]	Double transverse		25	0	(15/25 minor; 3/25 severe;)	(2/25) 8 abscess		(25/25) 100; (4/25 severe)
Johnson (1984)[24]	Transverse	101	67	0	50 (1 severe)	14	9	50; 35 severe
Whitmore (1984)[27]	Elliptical	25	17	0	(4/17) 24 (2 severe)	(4/17) 24	(4/17) 24	(13/17) 76; (1/17 severe)

Table 12.17. Morbidity of inguinal lymph node dissection

Is the morbidity of ilio-inguinal node dissection still prohibitive?

The main objection to early systematic node dissection has been that the morbidity and mortality is unacceptable, and that the surgery is likely to kill as many patients as potentially may be saved. Current surgical techniques have significantly reduced the morbidity, however (Table 12.17). The Gibson incision has a low incidence of necrosis, and plastic reconstruction may reduce this to negligible levels. Other techniques of reducing the morbidity include the Catalona modified and economic dissections. Early systematic dissection has a lower rate of complication than when it is done as a delayed procedure, which is further evidence in favour of early surgery. Hence, using modern techniques, the morbidity of node dissection should be low and the mortality zero.

Does radiotherapy have any place in the management of positive lymph nodes?

Radiotherapy in these circumstances is not curative (Table 12.18) as patients with positive nodes have a poor response to radiotherapy in terms of 5-year survival. Nevertheless, radiotherapy may have a place in the palliation of inoperable inguinal nodes, and in patients with positive pelvic lymph nodes. These patients do poorly with surgery,[13] and radiotherapy is one of the few options left open to them.

Reference	No. of patients	Stage	Five-year survival*	
			Radiotherapy	Surgery
McDougal (1986)[20]	5	III N+	0/5 (0)	
Fraley (1985)[17]	9	III N+	1/3 (33)	4/6 (67)
El-Demiry (1984)[28]	14	N+ve	2/8 (25)	4/6 (67)
Narayana (1982)[14]	23	N+	1/16 (6)	3/31 (10)

*Percentages in parentheses.

Table 12.18. Results of radiotherapy/surgery for positive nodes

Conclusions

Lymph node surgery has a critical role in the management of carcinoma of the penis. Given the incidence of this disease in developing countries, it has a major impact on health care in those areas. It is essential, therefore, to continue to study the results of surgery, and to pursue better and less morbid methods of treatment.

References

1. Jackson S M. The treatment of carcinoma of the penis. Br J Surg 1966; 53: 33–35
2. TNM classification of malignant tumours, 2nd ed. Geneva: Imprimerie G. de Buren S.A., 1974
3. Union Internationale Contre le Cancer (UIC): TNM atlas: Illustrated guide to the TNM/pTNM Classification of malignant tumours, 3rd ed. New York: Springer-Verlag, 1989: 237–244
4. Persky L. Epidemiology of cancer of the penis. Recent Results Cancer Res. 1977; 60: 97–109
5. Cancer epidemiology centre, Anti Cancer Council of Victoria, 1994
6. Bouchot O, Auvigne J, Peuvrel P et al. Management of regional lymph nodes in carcinoma of the penis. Eur Urol 1989; 16: 410–415
7. Kuruvilla J R, Garlick F H, Mammen K E. Results of surgical treatment of carcinoma of the penis. Aust N Z J Surg 1971; 41: 157–159
8. Ravi R. Morbidity following groin dissection for penile carcinoma. Br J Urol 1993; 72: 941–945
9. Orneallas A A, Seixas A L, Marota A et al. Surgical treatment of invasive squamous cell carcinoma of the penis: Retrospective analysis of 350 cases. J Urol 1994; 151: 1244–1249
10. Riveros M, Gorostiaga R. Cancer of the penis. Arch Surg 1962; 85: 377–383
11. Solsona E, Iborra I, Ricos J V et al. Corpus cavernosum invasion and tumor grade in the prediction of lymph node condition in penile carcinoma. Eur Urol 1992; 22: 115–118
12. Horenblas S, van Tinteren H, Delemarre J F M et al. Squamous cell carcinoma of the penis: accuracy of tumor, nodes and metastasis classification system, and role of lymphangiography, computerized tomography scan and fine needle aspiration cytology. J Urol 1991; 146: 1279–1283
13. Srinivas V, Morse M J, Herr H W et al. Penile cancer: relation of extent of nodal metastasis to survival. J Urol 1987; 137: 880–882
14. Narayana A S, Olney L E, Loening S A, Weimar G W, Culp D A. Carcinoma of the penis. Analysis of 219 cases. Cancer 1982; 49: 2185–2191
15. Nelson R P, Derrick F C, Allen W R. Epidermoid carcinoma of the penis. Br J Urol 1982; 54: 172–175
16. Young M J, Reda D J, Waters W B. Penile carcinoma: a twenty-five-year experience. Urology 1991; 38: 528–532
17. Fraley E E, Zhang G, Sazama R, Lange P H. Cancer of the penis. Prognosis and treatment plans. Cancer 1985; 55: 1618–1624
18. Pettaway C A, Stewart D, Vuitch F et al. Penile squamous carcinoma: DNA flow cytometry versus histopathology for prognosis. J Urol 1991; 145: 367A (abstr 618)
19. Fraley E E, Zhang G, Manivel C, Niehans G A. The role of ilioinguinal lymphadenectomy and significance of histological differentiation in treatment of carcinoma of the penis. J Urol 1989; 142: 1478–1482
20. McDougal W S, Kirchner F K Jr, Edwards R H, Killion L T. Treatment of carcinoma of the penis: the case for primary lymphadenectomy. J Urol 1986; 136: 38–41
21. Johnson D E, Lo R K. Management of regional lymph nodes in penile carcinoma. Five-year results following therapeutic groin dissections. Urology 1984; 24: 308–311

22. Johnson D E, Fuerst D E, Ayala A G. Carcinoma of the penis: experience with 153 cases. Urology 1973; 1: 404

23. Catalona W J. Modified inguinal lymphadenectomy for carcinoma of the penis with preservation of saphenous veins: technique and preliminary results. J Urol 1988; 140: 306–310

24. Assimos D G, Jarow J P. Role of laparoscopic pelvic lymph node dissection in the management of patients with penile cancer and inguinal adenopathy. J Endourol 1994; 8: 365–369

25. Maiche A G, Pyrhonen S, Karkinen M. Histological grading of squamous cell carcinoma of the penis: a new scoring system. Br J Urol 1991; 67: 522–526

26. Ornellas A A, Seixas A L C, de Moraes J R. Analyses of 200 lymphadenectomies in patients with penile carcinoma. J Urol 1991; 146: 330–332

27. Whitmore W F Jr, Vagaiwala M R. A technique of ilioinguinal lymph node dissection for carcinoma of the penis. Surg Gynecol Obstet 1984; 159: 573–578

28. El-Demiry M I M, Oliver R T D, Hope-Stone H F, Blandy J P. Reappraisal of the role of radiotherapy and surgery in the management of carcinoma of the penis. Br J Urol 1984; 56: 724–728

13

New approach in the treatment of penile carcinoma

N. Rodrigues Netto Jr
C. A. Levi D'Ancona

Introduction

Carcinoma of the penis, although uncommon, accounts for a significant proportion of genitourinary cancers in men. Management of the regional lymph nodes in these patients is controversial. Information about the regional node status is necessary for the appropriate management and cure of penile cancer.

The classical approach is to treat the primary tumour followed by 4 weeks of antibiotic therapy. Where the lymph nodes are not palpable after therapy, no further operation is recommended, but 20% have microscopic node invasion and consequently the treatment is compromised.[1] However, if the lymph nodes are still enlarged a radical lymphadenectomy is performed; as 50% have no tumour, patients are overtreated. Radical lymphadenectomy has a 30–50% incidence of major complications, including debilitating lymphoedema and skin flap necrosis, as well as a 30% mortality rate.[1]

To overcome these disadvantages, other techniques, such as sentinel node biopsy, have been developed, but biopsy of the sentinel node proved to be unreliable because of false-negative results.[2] Another procedure is fine needle aspiration cytology, which shows sampling errors in patients with multiple nodes measuring less than 2 cm.[3] A conservative (economic) inguinal lymphadenectomy is reported to reduce the inconvenience of radical lymphadenectomy.[1,4]

The authors propose that the primary tumour should be treated while at the same time a bilateral conservative lymphadenectomy is performed.

Patients and methods

Eight patients were treated by conservative lymphadenectomy plus penile surgery depending on the extent of the primary lesion.

The operation begins with a 10 cm incision approximately 2 cm medial and parallel to the femoral arterial pulse. The incision is deepened to the level of the Scarpa fascia. The adipose and lymphatic tissue deeper than the Scarpa fascia are removed en bloc. Therefore, the upper dissection margin is the inguinal ligament, the lateral margin is the medial margin of the saphenous and femoral veins and the medial margin is the adductor muscles (Fig. 13.1). When the frozen section shows negative lymph nodes, surgery is terminated. However, if the lymph nodes are positive, radical inguinal lymphadenectomy is performed. The economic lymphadenectomy is performed bilaterally, before penectomy. Iliac lymph node dissection is not performed.

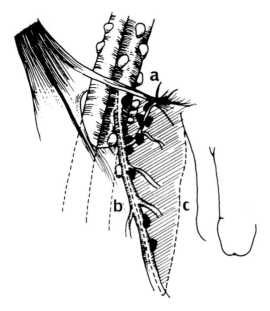

Figure 13.1. Margins of dissection of the lymph nodes: (a) inguinal ligament; (b) medial margin of the saphenous and femoral veins; (c) adductor muscles.

Results

Of the eight patients, two had histologically involved nodes, one bilateral and the other unilateral, and they were subjected to a radical inguinal lymphadenectomy. Two patients had mild oedema in the early postoperative period. At a 3-month follow-up, the patient subjected to the economic lymphadenectomy was free from lymphocoele and from oedema of the scrotum and lower limbs.

Discussion

A 4-week delay for a course of antibiotic therapy between penectomy and lymphadenectomy increases the treatment time and the total cost.

As some of the authors' patients live in remote areas, 30% of the follow-up is missed. The results do not show any increase in wound infection, as confirmed by 115 patients submitted to radical inguinal lymphadenectomy.[5]

Surgical staging is necessary to avoid over- and undertreatment, as these are frequent discrepancies between clinical assessment and pathological findings. Conservative lymphadenectomy, performed in eight patients, showed a small number of complications without inguinal recurrence.[6] This result was confirmed in another 29 patients (Table 13.1)[1,4]

The incidence of iliac node involvement is very low. In 130 patients undergoing radical lymphadenectomy, 60 showed positive inguinal lymph nodes and 14 (10.8%) positive iliac nodes. Only four (3%) had iliac metastases without inguinal nodes.[5] After 36 radical lymphadenectomies, 305 iliac lymph nodes examined overall did not show metastatic invasion of the iliac nodes.[4] These results justify the inguinal lymph node dissection. Resection of the iliac lymph nodes is not performed because, in the authors' opinion, when these nodes are positive the operation is palliative and it is not possible to control the disease surgically. Only in the case of a protocol to study the response of penile cancer to chemotherapy is this approach justifiable; otherwise there is no change in the patient's life expectancy.

In the authors' opinion, conservative inguinal lymph node dissection can be employed for surgical staging of the penile cancer at the same time as the treatment of the primary lesion.

	Complication rate (%)	
Complication	Radical (n = 101)	Conservative (n = 29)
Skin necrosis	50	0
Lymphoedema	15	0
Seroma	35	6.8
Wound infection	14	3.4
Lymphocoele	9	6.8
Thrombophlebitis	6	0
Bleeding	2	0
Scrotal oedema	15	0
Total	18.25	2.12

Table 13.1. Morbidity of radical and conservative lymphadenectomy

References

1. Catalona W J. Modified inguinal lymphadenectomy for carcinoma of the penis with preservation of saphenous veins: technique and preliminary results. J Urol 1988; 140: 306–310
2. Perinetti E P, Crane D B, Catalona W J. Unreliability of sentinal lymph node biopsy for staging penile carcinoma. J Urol 1980; 124: 734–735
3. Ayyappan K, Ananthakrishnan A, Sankaran V. Can regional lymph nodes involvement be predicted in patients with carcinoma of the penis? Br J Urol 1994; 73: 549–553
4. Costa R P, Schaal C H, Cortez J P. Nova proposta de limfadenectomia para o câncer do pênis: resultados preliminares. J Bras Urol 1989; 15: 242–246
5. Ornellas A A, Seixas A L C, Moraes J R. Analyses of 200 lymphadenectomies in patients with penile carcinoma. J Urol 1991; 146: 330–332
6. Rodrigues Netto N Jr, Levi D'Ancona C A L, Lopes A et al. Câncer de pênis — discussão anatomoclínica. J Bras Urol 1991; 17: 263–266

14

Lymphadenectomy for cancer of the penis

G. Pizzocaro   L. Piva   N. Nicolai

Introduction

Carcinoma of the penis mainly metastasizes via the lymphatic system. Metastases usually occur to regional lymph nodes by lymphatic embolization, rarely as a process of lymphatic permeation. The regional lymph nodes for carcinoma of the penis are the superficial, the deep inguinal, and the pelvic nodes, particularly those located in the obturator fossa. Approximately 20% of patients with metastases in more than one inguinal node also have pelvic nodal involvement.[1] Pelvic metastases in the absence of inguinal involvement are exceptionally rare.[2] Metastases to the common iliac and para-aortic nodes are considered to be distant metastases.

Although half of the patients present with enlarged inguinal nodes at diagnosis, less than 30% actually have nodal metastases. Regional metastases will develop during the follow-up in another 10–15% of category N_0 cases. Corpora cavernosa invasion and tumour grade have been related to the occurrence of nodal metastases.[1,3–6]

Involvement of inguinal nodes may be assessed by direct palpation, but palpable nodes are found to be cancerous in only about 60% of cases and clinically normal nodes contain unsuspected metastases in approximately 10–15% of cases.[7] Fine-needle aspiration cytology (FNAC) may add very useful information in the presence of palpable inguinal nodes. In the event of enlarged nodes and negative cytology, the patients should be re-examined 3–4 weeks after treatment of the primary tumour and adequate antimicrobial therapy, in order to allow inflammatory reactions to subside. Bipedal lymphangiography, CT of the abdomen and pelvis, or FNAC were found to be unable to detect regional lymph node invasion that has escaped clinical examination.[8] The authors do not use penile lymphangiography[9] or sentinel node biopsy[10,11] because the first procedure is difficult to perform and inguinal metastases have been reported following negative sentinel node biopsy.[12,13] Bipedal lymphangiography or CT scan of the abdomen and

Stage	Cancer of the penis
I	Tumour limited to the glans and/or prepuce
II	Tumour invading the shaft
III	Tumour with operable metastatic nodes
IV	Tumour invading adjacent structures, or with inoperable nodes or distant metastases

Table 14.1. Jackson's classification14 for cancer of the penis

Category	Classification	
	1978 edition[15]	1987 edition[16]
T_0	No evidence of primary tumour	Unchanged
T_{is}	Carcinoma in situ	Unchanged
T_a	Missing	Verrucous carcinoma
T_1	Strictly exophytic (<2 cm)	Invasion of subepithelial tissue
T_2	2–5 cm or minimal invasion	Invasion of corpora
T_3	>5 cm or deep invasion	Invasion of urethra or prostate
T_4	Invasion of adjacent structures	Unchanged
N_0	No evidence of regional node involvement	Unchanged
N_1	Involved moveable unilateral nodes	Metastases in a single superficial inguinal node
N_2	Involved moveable bilateral nodes	Multiple or bilateral superficial nodes
N_3	Fixed inguinal nodes	Metastases to deep inguinal or pelvic nodes
M_0	No evidence of distant metastases	Unchanged
M_1	Evidence of distant metastases	Unchanged
Regional nodes	Inguinal	Inguinal and pelvic

Table 14.2. UICC International TNM classification of penile cancer

pelvis may be of some help in detecting pelvic node invasion and in the determination of the extent of the disease in patients with unequivocal evidence of inguinal metastases.[8]

The most frequently used staging classifications for cancer of the penis are the Jackson's (Table 14.1)[14] and the UICC (Union Internationale Centre le Cancer) TNM system (Table 14.2).[15,16] Physical examination and imaging are minimum requirements to define N category. While the 1978 edition of the UICC international TNM classification[15] considered only the inguinal nodes as regional nodes, the 1987 edition[16] correctly considers the superficial, the deep inguinal, and the pelvic nodes as regional nodes, but the N category for fixed inguinal metastases has disappeared. Jackson's[14] and the 1987 UICC TNM[16] classifications are used in this chapter.

Lymphadenectomy for penile cancer

The management of regional lymph nodes in squamous-cell carcinoma of the penis is controversial.[17] The price to pay for a successful block dissection is high: delayed healing is common, and distressing lymphoedema of the lower limbs and external genitalia is a frequent late and permanent complication.[1,5,13,18] However, there is no evidence that radiotherapy is a satisfactory treatment for the inguinal nodes; the cure rate in patients with metastasis is extremely low, and prophylactic irradiation does not prevent the risk of subsequent metastases.[19] Surgical healing following unsuccessful radiotherapy is even more difficult.[20,21] At present, surgery remains the main therapy for nodal metastases in cancer of the penis. The authors' experience suggests that adjuvant and neoadjuvant chemotherapy may play a part in improving the long-term results of radical survey.[22]

Indications to lymphadenectomy

As only 30–50% of all patients with cancer of the penis will develop nodal metastases during the disease and the price to pay for a radical dissection is high, routine prophylactic lymphadenectomy cannot be recommended. However, the results of secondary lymphadenectomy in patients who develop nodal metastases during the follow-up have often been reported as unsatisfactory.[1,5,23] The aim is to select for nodal dissection those patients at a very high risk of harbouring nodal metastases. This risk increases significantly with the G grade[1,4,5] and invasion of the corpora.[3,6]

In the authors' experience,[24] nodal metastases occurred, at diagnosis or during the follow-up, in 21% of 129 T_1 patients, in 74% of 43 T_2 and in all eight T_3–T_4 patients. In category T_1, nodal metastases depended on G category — 10% in G_1, 30% in G_2 and in two of three in G_3. So far, concurrent penile amputation and lymphadenectomy are mandatory not only when there is obvious evidence of nodal involvement but also for the rare category T_3 and T_4 tumours. In addition, for the latter, en bloc surgery is recommended. Tumours invading the corpora are at very high risk of metastases, as well as the few G_3T_1 cases. The choice in these patients is between prophylactic lymphadenectomy or a very careful follow-up. Follow-up is indicated in the most frequent $G_{1-2}T_1(N_0)$ cases. It must be very carefully performed during the first 3 years, as nearly all metastases occur during this period.

Doubtful adenopathies should be re-evaluated a few weeks after treatment of the primary tumour following adequate antimicrobial therapy. The authors do not advise sentinel node biopsy,[10,11] because of frequent false-negative reports,[12,13] nor the Catalona's modified groin dissection,[25] because all patients suffered mild to moderate lower-limb oedema, and the dissection has been shown to be inadequate in patients with positive nodes.

Extension of the dissection and technical considerations

As reported previously, the regional nodes of cancer of the penis are the superficial and deep inguinal, the obturator and the external iliac nodes.[16] However, pelvic metastases do not usually occur in patients with negative inguinal nodes.[26] Conversly pelvic and bilateral nodal involvement are relatively frequent in patients with positive nodes[2,27] and their frequency increases with increasing metastatic spread.[1,26] A bilateral inguinopelvic lymphadenectomy is therefore indicated in patients with documented metastatic disease; in the event of a patient with doubtful inguinal nodes, the most suspect site should be operated on first. If inguinal nodes are negative, the other site can be carefully watched.

Whitmore's technique,[28] with two parainguinal incisions for the inguinal nodes and a separate suprapubic extraperitoneal approach for the pelvic nodes, is recommended for contemporary bilateral lymphadenectomy (Fig. 14.1). The authors prefer a longitudinal incision lateral to the femoral vessels for unilateral lymphadenectomy (Fig. 14.2). It can easily be extended upwards and, by dividing the inguinal ligament and abdominal muscles close to the superior iliac spine, the pelvic nodes can easily be reached on retracting the peritoneal sac medially.[29] Furthermore, as the major risk of inguinal lymphadenectomy is extensive skin necrosis with exposure of the femoral artery, it has been recommended that the femoral vessels are covered with the sartorius muscle.[4]

(a)

(b)

(c)

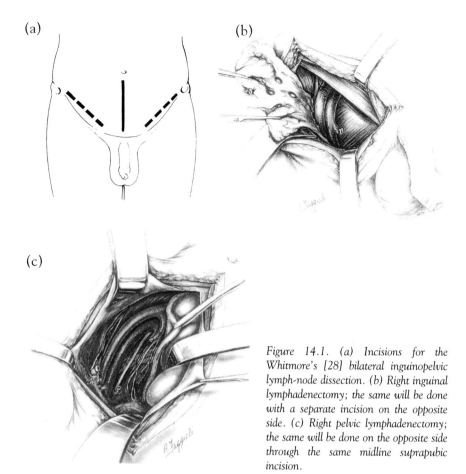

Figure 14.1. (a) Incisions for the Whitmore's [28] bilateral inguinopelvic lymph-node dissection. (b) Right inguinal lymphadenectomy; the same will be done with a separate incision on the opposite side. (c) Right pelvic lymphadenectomy; the same will be done on the opposite side through the same midline suprapubic incision.

Results of lymphadenectomy

Survival of patients with cancer of the penis has been mainly related to nodal involvement. Srivinas et al.[26] reported 85% disease-free survival following lymphadenectomy in 34 patients with negative nodes compared with 32% in 69 patients with positive histology who had not been lost to follow-up for at least 5 years. In addition, the extent of nodal involvement was important: patients with unilateral inguinal nodal metastases and neither extranodal tumour extension or iliac nodal involvement had a median 5-year survival rate of 56%. In particular, five of six patients with only one positive node survived disease free for over 5 years.

The management of regional lymph nodes according to tumour stage also seems to be important. None of the 19 Jackson stage I patients in

(a)

(b)

(c)

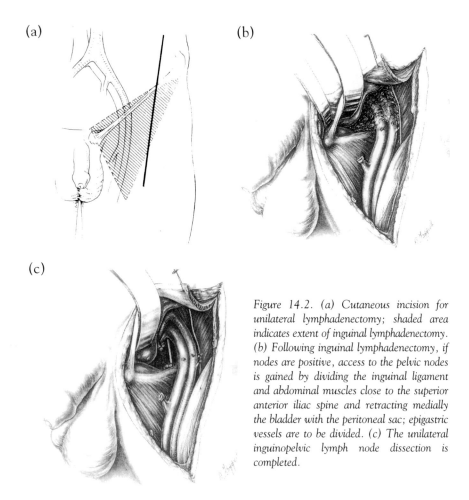

Figure 14.2. (a) Cutaneous incision for unilateral lymphadenectomy; shaded area indicates extent of inguinal lymphadenectomy. (b) Following inguinal lymphadenectomy, if nodes are positive, access to the pelvic nodes is gained by dividing the inguinal ligament and abdominal muscles close to the superior anterior iliac spine and retracting medially the bladder with the peritoneal sac; epigastric vessels are to be divided. (c) The unilateral inguinopelvic lymph node dissection is completed.

the series reported by McDougal et al.[13] had a lymph node dissection and none died of cancer. Of the nine patients with clinical stage II disease who had a groin dissection as part of the initial treatment (positive nodes in six), only one died of cancer, whereas nine of 14 stage II patients who initially had no lymphadenectomy died of the disease. Furthermore, the 5-year survival in 15 stage III patients submitted to lymphadenectomy was 67% compared with zero in eight unresected or irradiated patients. Similarly, Fraley et al.[5] reported no cancer-related death in 15 Jackson stage I patients treated with or without ileoinguinal lymphadenectomy, whereas in clinical stage II the 5-year disease-free survival was 100% in the nine patients with negative nodes, 75% in the eight patients with positive nodes, and only 15% in the 20 cases not initially treated with lymphadenectomy.

Recently, Horenblas[30] has statistically analysed several prognostic factors for survival in a series of 118 squamous-cell carcinomas of the penis treated between 1956 and 1989. Age group and type of treatment of the primary tumour were not statistically significant, in contrast with all the other factors. The 5-year (disease-specific) survival figures for T_1, T_2 and T_3 tumours (UICC 1978)[15] were 94, 59 and 52% respectively. A statistically significant survival difference was seen between patients with and without clinically suspected nodes. The 5-year survival figures according to the clinical N categories (UICC 1978)[15] were 93, 57, 50 and 17% for N_0, N_1, N_2 and N_3, respectively. Grade 3 tumours showed a statistically significant difference in 5-year survival compared with grade 1 tumours (47 and 79%, respectively). Cox's proportional hazard analysis showed that only N category and grade were highly statistically significant independent prognostic factors of survival.

Combined treatment modalities

Pre- and postoperative radiotherapy

As has been stated previously, prophylactic bilateral groin irradiation (50 Gy using mixed gamma rays and electron beams) is no longer recommended,[21] and preoperative irradiation leads to delayed healing, cutaneous sclerosis and lymphoedema.[20] In contrast. Gerbaulet and Lambin[21] advise postoperative irradiation for patients with extracapsular spread or multiple nodal metastases. The inguinal and iliac regions should be treated with a dose of 45–50 Gy in fractions of 2 Gy with cobalt of high-energy photons. Special skin care must be instituted to prevent moist epidermitis and serious discomfort to the patient. However, nowadays postoperative irradiation can be replaced by adjuvant chemotheraphy.

Adjuvant chemotherapy

Starting in 1979, the authors introduced vincristine, bleomycin and methotrexate (VBM) adjuvant chemotherapy (Table 14.3) for radically resected nodal metastases from squamous cell carcinoma of the penis.[22] The chemotherapy is administered at home with the cooperation of the family doctor. Patients are checked for toxicity in the outpatient department every 4 weeks. A total of 12 cycles are administered at weekly intervals. The therapy is relatively well tolerated; in the rare event of moderate myelotoxicity or mucositis it is delayed for a week. In elderly patients and in patients with chronic bronchitis, only one dose of

Drug	Dose
Vincristine	1 mg i.v. on day 1
Bleomycin	15 mg i.m. 6 and 24 h after vincristine[†]
Methotrexate	30 mg p.o. on day 3

*To be repeated weekly for 12 weeks
[†]In elderly patients and in patients with chronic bronchitis only the first bleomycin
dose is administered and methotrexate is anticipated on day 2.

Table 14.3. Vincristine, bleomycin and methotrexate (VBM) combination chemotherapy

bleomycin is administered. In the event of documented lung toxicity, bleomycin is withdrawn.

Between 1979 and 1990, 25 consecutive patients with radically resected nodal metastases from squamous cell carcinoma of the penis entered the adjuvant VBM protocol at the authors' institution.[24] All patients had a radical inguinopelvic lymph-node dissection and pelvic nodes were involved in seven cases. Only four (16%) patients relapsed, with a 5-year disease-free actuarial survival of 82%. These findings compare favourably with a previous series of 31 patients submitted to radical inguinopelvic lymph-node dissection alone, whose 5-year disease-free survival was only 37%. A more accurate analysis of these two series allowed some risk factors to be identified in patients with metastatic nodes.[24] In the series of 31 patients who did not receive adjuvant chemotherapy, bilateral nodal involvement, extracapsular spread, nodes larger than 2 cm, pelvic nodal involvement and more than one involved node were associated with poor prognosis, whereas in the series of 25 patients treated with adjuvant VBM, only bilaterality of metastases (and pelvic node involvement) remained significantly associated with poor prognosis ($p=0.006$). In particular, all four relapses occurred in the eight patients with bilateral nodal involvement. Furthermore, none of the nine patients who had solitary intranodal metastases suffered any relapse, independent of adjuvant chemotherapy. This small subset of patients seems to have no need for adjuvant chemotherapy, whereas patients with bilateral nodal involvement probably need a more aggressive adjuvant regimen.

Neoadjuvant chemotherapy for fixed inguinal nodes

Primary chemotherapy often meant palliation for unresectable metastases from squamous cell carcinoma of the penis, and it has been often associated with radiotherapy. Nevertheless, some important results have been obtained with primary chemotherapy in recent reports.[31–34] Considering together the experiences of Hussein,[31] Shammas,[32] Dexeus[33] and Kattan,[34] it is possible to consider a population of 29 patients who have been treated with various cisplatin combination chemotherapies for (primary or recurrent) fixed inguinal metastases from squamous cell carcinoma of the penis. Objective responses have been achieved in 19 (66%) cases, of whom 11 (38%) could be radically resected: 5 (17%) have been reported to be alive disease-free at 12, 24, 32, 32 and 57 months.[10–13]

The potential advantage of neoadjuvant chemotherapy in resectable inguinal metastases was evaluated by Fisher and associates in five patients with Jackson stage III squamous cell carcinoma of the penis.[35] Two courses of cisplatin plus fluorouracil (PF) combination chemotherapy (Table 14.4) were to be administered before inguinopelvic dissection. One patient, who was unresponsive to the first cycle, refused any further treatment and died of progressive disease. Four patients achieved an objective remission and underwent surgery: two had no viable tumour in the specimen and two had residual disease; one of them received postoperative radiotherapy. No relapse was recorded after a follow-up of 6–40 months. It is not known whether the two patients with negative nodes were complete responders to chemotherapy or there was a clinical staging error.

Since 1979, 16 consecutive patients with fixed nodal metastases from squamous cell carcinoma of the penis have been treated at the authors' institution with neoadjuvant chemotherapy.[24] The first 13 patients were to receive 12 weekly courses of VBM combination chemotherapy and the final three were to be treated with four courses of PF. Seven of the first 13 patients achieved a partial remission and underwent the operation, but only five could be radically resected. Two of these five

Drug	Dose[†]
Cisplatin	100 mg/m^2 i.v. on day 1 plus hydration and antiemetics
Fluorouracil	1 g/m^2/day for 96 h continous i.v. infusion, following cisplatin

*Every 21 days for two to four cycles.
[†]Dose/m^2 of patient's body surface area.

Table 14.4. Cisplatin and fluorouracil (PF) combination chemotherapy*

radically resected patients are alive and disease-free after 5 and 13 years, respectively; they represent 15% of the 13 patients treated with neoadjuvant VBM. The three patients who relapsed after radical surgery survived for 16, 27 and 32 months. Of the eight patients who were not rendered disease free, five died of progressive disease between 11 and 32 months, and three could receive second-line PF combination chemotherapy.

Of the six patients treated with PF (three previously treated with VBM and three naïve), five achieved a partial remission and underwent surgery, which was radical in four. Three of the four radically resected patients are alive and disease free after 3, 8 and 10 years, respectively. The remaining three patients survived for 3–10 months. Overall, 9 (56%) of 16 patients with fixed inguinal nodes could be radically resected following primary chemotherapy, and 5 (31%) have probably been cured. Cisplatin-based chemotherapy is probably to be preferred to VBM as first-line treatment for patients with fixed inguinal nodes.

Conclusions

Primary lymphadenectomy is mandatory in all patients with obvious evidence of resectable inguinal metastases from squamous cell carcinoma of the penis. As, in these patients, both pelvic and bilateral nodal involvement are relatively frequent, a bilateral inguinopelvic lymphadenectomy is indicated.

Doubtful inguinal nodes are to be re-evaluated a few weeks after treatment of the primary tumour with adequate antimicrobial therapy. If nodes persist and they are still doubtful, imaging and FNAC may be of little help, and inguinal lymphadenectomy is indicated on the most suspect site. If inguinal nodes are negative, it is not necessary to remove the pelvic nodes and the other site can be carefully watched.

It seems that all T_3 and T_4 tumours are associated with metastases. So far, bilateral inguinopelvic lymph node dissection is indicated in all these cases, and lymphadenectomy should be performed en bloc with the primary tumour in the case of a T_4 cancer.

In clinical T_1–$T_2 N_0$ patients, the risk of developing nodal metastases is significantly associated with invasion of corpora (T_2) and/or high grade (G_3). These patients must be very carefully followed for the first 3 years, or, alternatively, they have to undergo prophylactic lymphadenectomy, in spite of the risk of developing postoperative leg oedema.

The survival of patients with penile cancer mainly depends on nodal metastases: it is excellent in patients with negative nodes, whereas the

5-year survival is approximately 40% in patients with radically resected nodal metastases. This relatively poor prognosis of patients with radically resected nodal metastases can be transformed into a 5-year expected disease-free survival of approximately 80% with VBM adjuvant chemotherapy. Only patients with bilateral nodal involvement probably need a more aggressive adjuvant treatment.

Unresectable nodal metastases from squamous cell carcinoma of the penis is a challenging issue. Nevertheless, combination chemotherapy appears to be able to achieve major responses in approximately two-thirds of patients, resectability in about 50%, and durable disease-free survival in 15–30%. Of the two reported regimens (Table 14.3 and 14.4), VBM is the easiest to administer but, probably, is also the weakest. At present, the authors believe that the PF regimen is advisable as first-line therapy in patients with fixed inguinal nodes or advanced disease.

Last but not least, the authors emphasize that occasional patients treated in the neoadjuvant setting for 'resectable' nodal metastases progressed to unresectability during the therapy, and that no patient with metastatic disease was definitely cured with chemotherapy alone.[31–35] To date, radical surgery remains the milestone to achieve a definite cure in patients with nodal metastases from squamous cell carcinoma of the penis, while combination chemotherapy is expected to improve the cure rate.

References

1. Horenblas S, Van Tinteren H, Delamarre J F M et al. Squamous cell carcinoma of the penis—III. Treatment of regional lymphnodes. J Urol 1993; 149: 492–497
2. Riveros M, Gorostiaga R. Cancer of the penis. Arch Surg 1962; 85: 377–382
3. Crawford E D, Dawkins C A. Cancer of the penis. In: Skinner D G, Lieskovsky G (eds) Diagnosis and management of genitourinary cancer. Philadelphia: Saunders, 1988: 549–563
4. Blandy J P. Carcinoma of the penis. In: Veronesi U (ed) Surgical oncology. Berlin: Springer-Verlag, 1989; 746–755
5. Fraley E E, Zhang G, Manuvel C, Niehans G A. The role of ileo-inguinal lymphadenectomy and significance of histological differentiation in treatment of carcinoma of the penis. J Urol 1989; 142: 1478–1482
6. Solsona E, Jborra J, Ricos J V et al. Corpus cavernosum invasion and tumor grade in the prediction of lymphnode metastases. Eur Urol 1992; 22: 115–118
7. Persky L, deKernion J. Carcinoma of the penis. CA 1986; 36: 258–273
8. Horenblas S, Van Tinteren H, Delamarre J F M et al. Squamous cell carcinoma of the penis: accuracy of tumor nodes and metastases classification system, and role of lymphangiography, computed tomography scan and fine needle aspiration cytology. J Urol 1991; 146: 1279–1283
9. Kuisk H. Penile lymphography. In: Green W H (ed) Technique of lymphography. St, Louis: I.N.C., 1971; 135–140

10. Cabanas R M. An approach for the treatment of penile carcinoma. Cancer 1977; 39: 456–460

11. Cabanas R M. Anatomy and biopsy of sentinel lymphnodes. Urol Clin North Am 1992; 19: 267–276

12. Perinetti E, Crane D B, Catalona W T. Unreliability of sentinel lymphnode biopsy for staging penile carcinoma. J Urol 1980; 124: 734–735

13. McDougal W S, Kirchner F K, Edwards R H, Killion L T. Treatment of carcinoma of the penis: the case for primary lymphadenectomy. J Urol 1986; 136: 38–41

14. Jackson S M. Treatment of carcinoma of the penis. Br J Surg 1966; 53: 33–35

15. Harmer H, (ed) UICC TNM classification of malignant tumours, 3rd ed. Geneva: Buren S.A., 1978; 126–128

16. Hermaneck P, Sobi H (eds) UICC TNM classification of malignant tumours, 4th ed. Berlin: Springer-Verlag, 1987; 130–132

17. Abi-Aad A S, deKernion J B. Controversies in the ileoinguinal lymphadenectomy for cancer of the penis. Urol Clin North Am 1992; 19: 319–324

18. Ornellas A A, Correa Seixas A L, De Morales J R. Analysis of 200 lymphadenectomies in patients with penile carcinoma. J Urol 1991; 146: 330–332

19. Jones W G, Fossa S D, Harmers H, van den Bogaert W. Penis cancer: a review by the Joint Committee of the European Organization for Research and Treatment of Cancer (EORTC), Genito-urinary and Radiotherapy Groups. J Surg Oncol 1989; 40: 227–231

20. Gursel E D, Georgountros C, Uson A C et al. Penile cancer: clinicopathological study of 64 cases. Urology 1978; 1: 569–578

21. Gerbaulet A, Lambin P. Radiotherapy of cancer of the penis. Indications, advantages, pitfalls. Urol Clin North Am 1992; 19: 325–332

22. Pizzocaro G, Piva L. Adjuvant and neoadjuvant vincristine, bleomycin and methotrexate for inguinal metastases from squamous cell carcinoma of the penis. Acta Oncol 1988; 27: 823–824

23. Johnson D E, Lo R K. Management of regional lymph nodes in penile carcinoma: five-year results following therapeutic groin dissection. Urology 1984; 24: 308–311

24. Pizzocaro G, Piva L, Faustini M, Nicolai N. Indications for lymphadenectomy and adjuvant or neoadjuvant chemotherapy for lymph-node metastases from squamous-cell carcinoma of the penis. Proc 23rd SIU congr Sydney, 1994; 294 (abstr 805)

25. Catalona W. Modified inguinal lymphadenectomy for carcinoma of the penis with preservation of saphenous vein: technique and preliminary results. J Urol 1988; 140: 306–310

26. Srivinas V, Morse N J, Herr H W et al. Penile cancer: relation of extent of nodal metastases to survival. J Urol 1987; 137: 880–882

27. Livne P M, Pontes J E. Tumors of penis, scrotum and spermatic cord. In: Graham S D Jr (ed) Urologic oncology. New York: Raven Press, 1986; 369–382

28. Whitmore W F, Vagaiwala M R. A technique of ileoinguinal lymph node dissection for carcinoma of the penis. Surg Gynecol Obstet 1984; 573–578

29. Pizzocaro G. I tumori dell'apparato genitale maschile. In: Veronesi U (ed) Trattato di chirurgia oncologica. Turin: UTET, 1989; 571–618

30. Horenblas S. The management of penile squamous cell carcinoma a retrospective and prospective study. Thesis, Universiteit van Amsterdam, BV Export drukkerij, Zoetermeer, 1993; 145–160

31. Hussein A M, Benedetto P, Sridar K S. Chemotherapy with cisplatin and 5-fluorouracil for penile and urethral squamous cell carcinoma. Cancer 1990; 433: 65

32. Shammas F V, Ous S, Fossa S D. Cisplatin and 5-fluorouracil and advanced cancer of the penis. J Urol 1992; 630: 147

33. Dexeus F H, Logothetis C J, Sella A et al. Combinations chemotherapy with methotrexate, bleomycin and cisplatin for advanced squamous cell carcinoma of the male genital tract. J Urol 1991; 1284: 146

34. Kattan J, Culine S, Droz J P et al. Penile cancer chemotherapy: twelve years' experience at Institut Gustave-Roussy. Urology 1993; 559: 42

35. Fisher H A G, Barada J H, Horton J, von Roemeling R. Noeadjuvant therapy with cisplatin and 5-fluorouracil for stage III squamous cell carcinoma of the penis. J Urol 1990; 143: 352A (abstr 653)

Testis

VI

Role of retroperitoneal lymphadenectomy (RLND) when patients with non-seminomatous germ cell testicular tumours are at high risk of needing lymph node surgery plus chemotherapy

15

D. A. Swanson

Introduction

At the University of Texas M. D. Anderson Cancer Center, there has been a long-standing interest in the role of retroperitoneal lymphadenectomy (RLND) in the management of non-seminomatous germ cell testicular tumours (NSGCTT). History has shown this role to be a dynamic one, changing while seeking to provide more efficient therapy to patients with this disease. It has been the Center's approach over the years constantly to monitor the experience and, when the data suggest a potentially better approach, to formulate a hypothesis and make the appropriate change in treatment policy. The policy is then re-evaluated to see if it is, indeed, better than the old one. Data are now available that enable two relatively recent changes in treatment policy for NSGCTT to be reviewed; those data and the author's conclusions are presented in this chapter.

Background

To understand the changes, it is necessary to review briefly the history of management of NSGCTT at M. D. Anderson. In October 1981, two protocols for patients with NSGCTT were instituted — surveillance for all patients with clinical stage I disease, and initial chemotherapy (as opposed to RLND) for all patients with clinical stage II disease.

The rationale for surveillance was based on the observations and early clinical experience of Dr Michael Peckham and his colleagues at the Royal Marsden Hospital.[1] Initially, any patient with clinical stage I disease who had no evidence of metastases on physical exam or on chest radiography, CT scan or bipedal lymphangiogram, and who had normal serum-α-foetoprotein (AFP) and β-chain human chorionic gonadotrophin levels, was eligible for surveillance. The data from the first 99 unselected patients are now very mature (a median follow-up of 81 months; 83% had at least 60 months of follow-up, and 94% at least 36 months) and have been published.[2] Twenty-seven patients (27%) 'relapsed', i.e. manifested clinically occult and previously unrecognized metastases in the lungs or retroperitoneum, or had rising serum biomarkers. However, because these patients were not selected, except to exclude those with definite evidence of metastatic disease, this relapse rate was not surprising.

Several prognostic factors were identified in the mid-1980s that helped to predict which patients with stage I NSGCTT might have occult metastases and be at high risk to 'relapse' and require further therapy. The most important of these factors were some histological types, particularly high-volume embryonal carcinoma and low-volume teratoma, and lymphatic and vascular invasion.[3–6] Several investigators also reported that if more than one risk factor were present, the chance of relapse or the chance of finding positive lymph nodes at the time of RLND was substantially higher.[5,7] At the author's own institution, the records were examined of 82 patients with clinical stage I NSGCTT who were treated by observation alone following radical orchiectomy and in whom there were records of both a complete histopathological evaluation and preorchiectomy serum AFP levels.[8] Analysis of these data showed the patients were at low risk if they had less than 80% embryonal carcinoma in the primary tumour, if their preorchiectomy AFP was less than 80 ng/dl (by any of various assays, because many were performed at other institutions), and if there was no vessel (vascular or lymphatic) invasion. Patients were considered to be at high risk if any one of these factors was present. Of the 30 patients considered to be at low risk using these three risk criteria, not a single patient relapsed, whereas 24 of the 52 high-risk patients (46%) did relapse ($p < 0.00001$). Thus, it is clear that it is possible to identify patients who are at very low risk, at intermediate risk, and at high risk for relapse following radical orchiectomy for clinical stage I NSGCTT.

The second major protocol that was begun in October 1981 recommended initial chemotherapy for all patients with clinical stage II NSGCTT. The rationale for this approach was that these patients were at high risk for subsequent relapse despite lymphadenectomy, and that primary chemotherapy by itself might control the disease in some patients and reduce the number who required both RLND and chemotherapy. The data demonstrated that the presence or absence of teratomatous elements in the primary tumour had a profound influence on whether chemotherapy alone would be sufficient, or whether patients would require an RLND for a residual mass after chemotherapy. Patients were far more likely to require RLND after chemotherapy if their primary tumour had embryonal carcinoma plus teratoma (10/29, 34.5%) than if it had embryonal carcinoma without any teratomatous elements (3/31, 9.7%).[9] It was also found that although the relapse rates were similar among 64 high-risk patients whether teratoma was present (41%) or not (54%), fewer patients relapsed above the diaphragm if teratoma was present (4/21) than if it was not (6/7).

These parallel observations led the author and colleagues to change the approach to the management of patients with clinical stage I or stage II NSGCTT. Starting in mid-1988, it was recommended that patients with clinical stage I disease who were at high risk of relapse — those with at least 80% embryonal carcinoma in their primary tumour, a preorchiectomy AFP greater than 80 ng/dl, or vascular or lymphatic invasion, particularly if they had teratoma in their primary tumour — should undergo initial RLND, in the hope of sparing some patients the disappointment of relapse as well as the potential risk of delaying therapy. In the hope, also, of decreasing the need for both RLND and chemotherapy in some patients with clinical stage II disease, starting in 1985 initial RLND was recommended for stage II patients whose primary tumour contained teratoma. It is now possible to evaluate these two new policies and make some conclusions as to their efficacy.

Initial RLND for high-risk stage I

From 1 September 1988 until 30 June 1993, initial RLND was performed on 24 patients with clinical stage I disease at high risk of subsequent relapse. Patients were at high risk by virtue of having at least 80% embryonal carcinoma (nine patients), AFP of more than 80 ng/dl (16 patients) and vascular or lymphatic invasion (nine patients); ten patients had two risk factors. RLND revealed lymph node metastases in six of these 24 patients (25%). Of the patients who were determined by RLND to have positive lymph nodes, four were at high risk by virtue of at least 80% embryonal carcinoma (Table 15.1). In fact, of the nine patients who had at least 80% embryonal carcinoma, four did have positive lymph nodes.

No. of Patients	Risk factors
2	≥ 80% embryonal
1	AFP > 80 ng/dl
1	≥ 80% embryonal plus AFP > 80ng/dl
1	≥ 80% embryonal plus vessel invasion
1	AFP > 80 ng/dl plus vessel invasion

Table 15.1. Risk factors present in stage I NSGCTT patients determined by RLND to have positive lymph nodes

Unfortunately, following RLND, relapses occurred in eight of the 24 patients, only two of whom had had positive lymph nodes. The lungs were the site of relapse in six patients (only one had had positive lymph nodes), suprahilar lymph nodes were involved in one patient (his RLND had revealed 11 of 69 lymph nodes to be positive), and rising serum markers indicated relapse in one patient (who had had negative lymph nodes). Thus, two of the six patients who had had positive lymph nodes had relapses, one in the lungs and one in suprahilar lymph nodes, and six of the 18 patients with negative lymph nodes had relapses, five in the lungs and one with rising serum markers.

All relapsing patients received chemotherapy; seven are known to be alive without any evidence of disease after a median follow-up of 22 months (range 12–42 months), and one patient was lost to follow-up at 33 months.

Only four patients had positive lymph nodes and did not relapse after a median follow-up of 41 months (range 29–59 months). They are the only patients potentially cured by RLND and it is entirely possible that delayed RLND (i.e. RLND when retroperitoneal relapse was identified) might also have been curative.

Twelve of the patients who had negative lymph nodes upon RLND have not revealed any additional tumour after a median follow-up of 31 months (range 5–60 months). If they had been on surveillance instead of undergoing initial RLND, they should not have required any therapy after orchiectomy. In these patients, RLND might be considered to have been unnecessary.

These results suggest that surveillance for patients with stage I disease at high risk of relapse might still be more appropriate than initial RLND. Under surveillance, if a patient demonstrated relapse as visceral metastases, he would obviously require chemotherapy and would subsequently undergo RLND or other surgery only if he had a residual mass. If he relapsed in the retroperitoneum, a delayed RLND might be curative (and since this high-risk group would be followed quite closely, it is unlikely that the retroperitoneal mass would be very large, which would reduce his risk of subsequent relapse outside the retroperitoneum). If he relapsed with rising serum markers only, delayed RLND would also be recommended although this group of patients stands at significant risk of subsequently manifesting disease outside the retroperitoneum and might, anyway, require chemotherapy.

If this group of 24 patients had been placed on a surveillance protocol instead of undergoing initial RLND, the number of patients who required RLND plus chemotherapy would undoubtedly have been markedly less (Table 15.2). For patients who received chemotherapy for metastases outside the retroperitoneum, some might not have required RLND, although a few patients, obviously, would have required both anyway; this number is estimated to be two or three, based on the author's experience. Thus, instead of all 24 patients getting an RLND initially, an estimated six patients would under RLND if surveillance were practised, even though the patient was at high risk, and an estimated eight patients would eventually require chemotherapy, a number no different from the eight patients in this series who did receive chemotherapy. The greatest difference is that as few as two patients would require both RLND and chemotherapy in a surveillance protocol, whereas eight patients in this series were treated by both.

It is concluded that patients with high-risk clinical stage I NSGCTT are not necessarily helped by initial RLND, except to secure the retroperitoneum and make diagnosis and treatment of relapse potentially easier. RLND does not, however, decrease the need for chemotherapy in this high-risk group, and initial RLND leads to an increased number of patients who require both RLND plus chemotherapy compared with

Treatment	Initial RLND	Surveillance
None	0	12
RLND alone	16	4
RLND + CTX*	8	2
CTX alone	0	6

*Chemotherapy.

Table 15.2. Comparison of treatment modalities eventually required for stage I NSGCTT patients undergoing initial RLND versus surveillance

patients on surveillance. In the author's opinion, optimum therapy for this group of patients has not yet been defined, and a protocol of surveillance alone versus two courses of pre-emptive chemotherapy and close observation is currently being evaluated. An alternative approach might recommend RLND for this group of patients plus two courses of adjuvant chemotherapy, but this has the disadvantage of guaranteeing the morbidity of both RLND and chemotherapy, even if the morbidity of two courses of chemotherapy is less than that of full-dose chemotherapy for metastatic disease.

Initial RLND for stage II

The author's rationale for recommending initial RLND for patients with clinical stage II NSGCTT was that this might decrease the need for both RLND plus chemotherapy in some patients, particularly if their primary tumour contained teratomatous elements. From January 1985 to August 1993, initial RLND was performed on 34 such patients and these results now permit a clear conclusion.

RLND reveal metastatic disease in the retroperitoneal lymph nodes in all 20 patients who had definite radiographic evidence of a mass, and in eight of the nine patients who had only persistently elevated serum markers; none of the five patients who had equivocal findings in the retroperitoneum on either CT scan or bipedal lymphangiogram had positive lymph nodes. Twenty-one patients are alive without evidence of disease after a median follow-up of 45 months since RLND (range 9–97 months) without having required additional therapy. Thirteen patients (38%) relapsed after RLND and required chemotherapy for their visceral metastases (four patients), supraclavicular or pelvic lymph node metastases (three patients), or rising serum markers (six patients, three of whom never achieved normal serum markers after RLND). Several risk factors did seem influential: relapses occurred in ten of the 11 patients (91%) who had at least five positive lymph nodes, six of the seven patients (86%) who had vascular or lymphatic invasion, and two of the five patients (40%) who had a retroperitoneal mass at least 4 cm in diameter on CT scan. All 13 patients are alive without evidence of disease after a median follow-up of 45 months (range 17–68 months) after chemotherapy.

During this same interval, 75 additional patients received initial chemotherapy for stage II NSGCTT, 24 of whom had teratomatous elements in their primary tumour, but who were not sent for initial RLND for various reasons. Nine of these 24 patients (37.5%) required RLND after initial chemotherapy, confirming the author's earlier published findings.[9]

The data show that RLND alone cures some patients with clinical stage II NSGCTT who have teratoma, but that many require chemotherapy afterwards. In the present series, this proportion was 38% of the patients, a rate virtually identical to that of patients with teratoma who eventually required RLND for a residual mass after initial chemotherapy (Table 15.3). Thus, the data refute the author's hypothesis: initial RLND does not appear to decrease the number of patients who need both RLND plus chemotherapy. It is hoped that future studies will identify prognostic factors that will enable optimal initial therapy, i.e. either RLND or chemotherapy, to be selected rationally. In the meantime, however, because no increase was seen in the number of patients requiring double therapy after initial RLND, this approach is still recommended for patients with stage II NSGCTT because it prevents clinical overstaging; it is associated with reduced surgical morbidity compared with that seen with RLND after chemotherapy, particularly the potential for successful nerve-sparing; and relapse is easier to diagnose and treat when not in the retroperitoneum.

| | Percentage of patients receiving treatment | | |
Initial treatment	RLND Only	CTX Only	Both
RLND (present series)	62	0	38
CTX			
Old series[9]	0	65.5	34.5
Contemporary	0	62.5	37.5

Table 15.3. Treatment received by patients with clinical stage II NSGCTT by initial treatment

Conclusions

There are still many unanswered questions about the role of lymph node surgery in testis cancer. In the author's opinion, well-defined prognostic factors can identify some patients with clinical stage I NSGCTT at such low risk for relapse that they do not need RLND, no matter how low the morbidity. It is clear, however, that RLND does cure some patients with stage II disease, both those who are clinically stage I but pathologically stage II and some patients who present with clinical stage II disease. However, there remains a subset of patients who require both RLND plus chemotherapy for eradication of all disease, although it is hoped that selection of the right initial therapy, i.e. either RLND or chemotherapy, may keep this number to a minimum. The avoidance of double therapy seems to be a worthwhile goal, and further research on how to select initial therapy seems well worth pursuing. The role of adjuvant chemotherapy, particularly when given as only two courses, is still unknown but must be considered when investigators plan future studies to address these important questions.

References

1. Peckham M J, Husband J E, Barrett A *et al.* Orchidectomy alone in testicular stage I non-seminomatous germ-cell tumours. Lancet 1982; 2: 678–680

2. Swanson D A. The case for observation of patients with clinical stage I nonseminomatous germ cell testicular tumors. Semin Urol 1993; 92–98

3. Hoskin P, Dilly S, Easton D *et al.* Prognostic factors in stage I non-seminomatous germ-cell testicular tumours managed by orchiectomy and surveillance: implications for adjuvant chemotherapy. J Clin Oncol 1986; 4: 1031–1036

4. Sogani P C. Evolution of the management of stage I nonseminomatous germ-cell tumors of the testis. Urol Clin North Am 1991; 18: 561–573

5. Freedman L S, Jones W G, Peckham M J *et al.* Histopathology in the prediction of relapse of patients with stage I testicular teratoma treated by orchidectomy alone. Lancet 1987; 2: 294–298

6. Read G, Stenning S P, Cullen M H *et al.* Medical Research Council prospective study of surveillance for stage I testicular teratoma. J Clin Oncol 1992; 10: 1762–1768

7. Fung C Y, Kalish L A, Brodsky G L *et al.* Stage I nonseminomatous germ cell testicular tumor: prediction of metastatic potential by primary histopathology. J Clin Oncol 1988; 6: 1467–1473

8. Wishnow K I, Johnson D E, Swanson D A *et al.* Identifying patients with low-risk clinical stage I nomseminomatous testicular tumours who should be treated by surveillance. Urology 1989; 34: 339–343

9. Swanson D A, Logothetis C J. Primary chemotherapy for clinical stage II nonseminomatous testicular carcinoma. Adv Urol 1988; 1: 129–144

Is it possible to preserve antegrade ejaculation in retroperitoneal lymphadenectomy due to residaul masses after primary chemotherapy for testicular cancer?

16

E. Solsona   I Iborra-Juan   J. V. Ricós-Torrent
J. L. Monrós-Lliso   R. Dumont-Martinez
J. Casanova-Ramon   V. Guillem-Porta

Introduction

Five-year survival for testicular cancer has dramatically increased over the past 30 years from 60% to a current rate of over 90%.[1-4] This improvement has been due to the appropriate integration of effective chemotherapy and surgery, associated with the advent of CT scan and reliable serum tumour markers.

In the early stages, radical lymphadenectomy results in disease control in 80–100% of patients; however, ejaculation loss has been observed in most patients.[5-8] Modifying the surgical boundaries of the lymphadenectomy procedure has resulted in preservation of ejaculation in 74–88% of patients.[6,8-12] Recently, in the same group of patients and taking into account neuroanatomical studies of ejaculation mechanisms,[11,13-15] Donohue[16] and Jewett[17] were able to preserve sympathetic nerve fibres so that ejaculation remained in 90–100% of patients.

In patients with retroperitoneal residual masses after chemotherapy, however, lymphadenectomy produced a permanent loss of ejaculation in most of the patients reported.[11,18,19] One of the goals of the study reported here was, therefore, to avoid this complication.

Since 1987, aiming to preserve antegrade ejaculation in patients with retroperitoneal residual masses after chemotherapy, the authors have combined changes in the boundaries of surgery with preservation of sympathetic structures during lymphadenectomy.

Patients and methods

Since November 1987, 21 patients with testicular cancer and retroperitoneal residual masses with normal serum tumour markers after chemotherapy have undergone modified lymphadenectomy. The characteristics of these 21 patients are shown in Table 16.1.

Before lymphadenectomy, all patients received primary chemotherapy: six received PVB (cisplatin, vinblastine and bleomycin, four to seven courses (mean five courses); ten received BEP (bleomycin, etoposide and cisplatin), four or five courses (mean 4.2), two patients received PE (cisplatin and etoposide), four courses each, and three patients received four courses of PEI (cisplatin, etoposide and ifosfamide).

The modifications in the lymphadenectomy technique have attempted to preserve, first, both sympathetic trunks, exposing the trunk on the same side as the residual mass from the outset; this enables the

Mean age (years)	26.9 (15–46)*
Tumour site (right/left)	8/13
Pathology:	
Embryonal carcinoma	5
Teratocarcinoma	6
Mixed tumours[†]	8
Seminoma	2
Stage[‡]	
IIB	4
IIC	9
III	2
IV	6
No. of patients with elevated markers[§]	17

*Range in parentheses.
[†]Mixed tumors: six embryonal ca ± teratocarcinoma ± yolk sac sumour ± seminoma; Two teratocarcinoma ± seminoma.
[‡]Royal Marsden classification.
[§]Before chemotherapy.

Table 16.1. Details of 21 patients with testicular cancer and retroperitoneal residual masses after chemotherapy

postganglionic branches roots to be identified. The dissection of the contralateral trunk is avoided by not removing the contralateral lymphatic chain. If the residual mass is large and the contralateral lymphatic chain has to be removed, both lumbar trunks are initially displayed. Second, the superior hypogastric plexus is preserved, avoiding the aortic dissection from the inferior mesenteric artery to the interiliac area. Third, the postganglionic branches that join the lumbar trunks to the superior hypogastric plexus are preserved. These are identified, both on the right side, in the interaortocaval area, and on the left side, in the paraortic area.

The remaining lymphatic chains are removed, even if they are apparently not infiltrated, as well as the residual mass and sclerotic tissues.

When sympathetic structures are included either in the residual mass or in scelerotic areas, these modifications are not made and a more extended exeresis is performed.

Non-urethral semen emission due to either lack or seminal emission or retrograde ejaculation was considered to constitute loss of ejaculation.

Results

The distribution of the retroperitoneal masses before and after chemotherapy is summarized in Table 16.2. The mean size of the residual masses was 6.1 cm (range 3–16 cm); pathological findings are shown in Table 16.3. The five patients with residual carcinoma subsequently received further chemotherapy.

All sympathetic trunks were preserved apart from two. The hypogastric plexus was preserved in all patients; however, in seven a partial resection had to be performed beacuse of the presence of sclerotic tissue in the inframesenteric area of the aorta. The right postganglionic branches could be preserved, during interaortocaval dissection, in five patients with left testicular tumours and in one patient with a right testicular tumour. However, the left postganglionic nerves could never be preserved, because they were included in the residual mass or sclerotic tissues, during para-aortic dissection.

Overall, 17 of 21 (81%) patients reported normal antegrade ejaculation postoperatively. The ejaculated volume was evaluated in all patients before lymphadenectomy and in those patients with normal ejaculation after lymphadenectomy, with a mean of 3.7 ml (range 1.5–6.5 ml) and mean of 3.3 ml (range 1.5–7 ml) respectively, the difference not being statistically significant ($p > 0.05$). Currently, four patients have no antegrade ejaculation; the condition of these patients is summarized in Table 16.4.

Lymphatic chain	Masses			
	Before chemotherapy		After chemotherapy	
	Right*	Left*	Right	Left
Paracaval	5	–	3	–
Precaval	5	–	3	–
Interaortacaval	8	3	8	3
Preaortic				
Supramesenteric	–	7	–	3
Inframesenteric	–	–	–	–
Paraortic	–	13	–	12
Interiliac	–	–	–	–
Retrocrural	2	–	–	–
Total (patients)	8	13	8	13

*Right and left indicate primary tumour site.

Table 16.2. Distribution of retroperitoneal masses before and after chemotherapy

Pathological findings	No.**
Fibrosis/necrosis*	10 (47.6)
Teratoma[†]	6 (28.6)
Carcinoma[‡]	5 (23.8)

*Two patients residual lung masses.
**Percentages in parentheses.
[†]One patient with vena cava invasion, two with areas of embryonal carcinoma.
[‡]One patient with foci of mesenchymal differentiation.

Table 16.3. Pathology of residual masses in 21 patients

All residual masses were removed completely, apart from one in which the pathologist reported positive surgical margins with residual carcinoma.

After a mean follow-up of 28.9 months (range 6–76 months), two (9.5%) patients have relapsed. One patient with a positive margin on pathological examination of the residual mass, received three courses of

Findings	Patient no.			
	1	2	3	4
Pathology*	MT	TC	EC	TC
Site	Left	Left	Right	Left
Stage	IV	IIC	III	IV
Mass diamter (cm)	8	9	11	13
Mass distribution:				
Paracaval			Yes	
Interaortocaval		Yes	Yes	Yes
Preaortic	Yes	Yes		Yes
Paraortic	Yes	Yes		Yes
Mass pathology	Teratoma	Fibrosis	Carcinoma	Fibrosis
Chemotherapy:	PVB	PVB	BEP	PEI
No. of courses	5	4	4	4
Structures:				
Trunk (resection)	Yes	No	No	No
Branches (removal)	Yes	Yes	Yes	Yes
Hypogastric plexus (resection)**	Yes	Yes	Yes	Yes
Follow-up (months)	45	21	32	14

*MT: mixed tumor; TC: teratocarcinoma; EC: embryonal carcinoma.
**Partial resection.

Table 16.4. Findings in patients in whom ejaculation was lost

vinblastine, ifosfamide and cisplatin, but the tumour metastasized to the lung without evidence of retroperitoneal recurrence. In the other patient the recurrence occurred in the retroperitoneal dissecction area; in this patient, the pathological report on the residual mass was of a carcinoma with foci of mesenchymal differentiation; the cancer recurred 14 months after lymphadenectomy, when the pathological report was of a leiomyosarcomatous lesion. After 37 months this patient is free of disease, having undergone a negative second laparotomy 9 months after the recurrent tumour has been removed.

All patients but two (90.5%) are alive and free of tumour. One patient had a fatal recurrence in the lung, another died of a heart attack with no recurrence of cancer.

No differences were observed in loss of ejaculation in relation to the initial stages, between the location (side) of the primary tumour, tumour markers and residual mass distribution; however, there appears to be a difference in relation to the residual mass size, in that lack of ejaculation was found in four of five patients in whom the residual mass was greater than 7 cm in diameter, whereas it did not occur in those in whom it was less than 7 cm.

The morbidity associated with the lymphandectomy procedure is summarized in Table 16.5.

Morbidity	No. of patients
Operative mortality	0
Patch caval resection	2*
Nephrectomy	1
Partial nephrectomy	1†
Prolonged lymphorrhoea	1
Prolonged ileus	2

*One patient with thrombus and caval wall teratomatous infilatration.
†Because of polar renal artery injury.

Table 16.5. Morbidity associated with modified lymphadenectomy procedure

Discussion

The greater efficiency of the current chemotherapentic protocols gives rise, in most cases, to a well-encapsulated residual mass, permitting a surgical procedure that is able to preserve some of the sympathetic structures that control the ejaculation mechanism.

The importance of conservation of the sympathetic nerve trunks is shown by the fact that their bilateral removal resulted in permanent loss of ejaculation in 54% of patients, whereas unilateral damage led only to transient loss of ejaculation.[20] These trunks are located deep in the groove between the psoas muscle and vertebral column;[13,14,16,17] they are, therefore, infiltrated by residual masses or sclerotic tissues only rarely — on two occasions in the authors' experience. Nevertheless, they can be injured during division of the lumbar vessels; thus, they must be clearly identified at the outset.

Superior hypogastric plexus resection produces a loss of ejaculation in almost all patients;[14,20] conservation of this plexus has therefore been described as the keystone of preservation of ejaculation in patients with early stage cancer of the testis who underwent modified lymphadenectomy.[6,8–12] The possibility of preservation of the hypogastric plexus depends on the location of the residual mass and sclerotic areas; for this reason, a partial resection had to be made in seven patients, four of whom lost antegrade ejaculation.

The postganglionic branches are seldom preserved, as they run through the interaortocaval and para-aortic areas,[13,15–17] in which residual masses are most often located, in the authors' experience (Table 16.2) and that of Donohue.[21] Postganglionic nerves could be preserved during interaortocaval dissection, in five patients with a left testicular tumour where interaortocaval chains were not involved, and in one patient with a right testicular tumour because the mass was small and well encapsulated, enabling the right postganglionic branches to be preserved. However, the left postganglionic branches, could never be preserved during para-aortic dissection, owing to the presence of residual masses and sclerotic tissues in this area.

The four patients with loss of antegrade ejaculation had large residual masses (8, 9, 11 and 13 cm). Partial resection of the hypogastric plexus and removal of the postganglionic branches were performed in all these patients, and one of the sympathetic trunks was also removed in two patients. Ejaculation loss seems to be in relation to residual mass size: in this series all patients with masses less than 7 cm in maximum diameter preserved ejaculation, probably because the size of the tumour determines the possibility of preserving the sympathetic structures associated with the ejaculation mechanism.

With regard to retroperitoneal recurrence, in this series one patient had a recurrence in the retroperitoneal dissection area, without involving the retained lymphatic chains. This represents a local recurrence rate of 4.7%, similar to the 4.3% reported by Fossa,[1] who performed a more extended bilateral lymphadenectomy. However, the patient in question was a very exceptional case, probably relapsing because of incomplete resection of the residual mass, rather than because the surgical margins were not sufficiently extensive, since the recurrent mass was in the area dissected. In fact, in this series and in another carried out before 1987, the apparent healthy lymphatic chains removed displayed, sometimes, necrotic or scar tissue but never revealed any malignant or teratomatous lesion on pathologial examination. On the other hand, in this modified lymphadenectomy, the retained lymphatic chains were the area that showed a lower incidence of metastases, both in the initial evaluation of the patient[22,23] and in the distribution of residual masses after chemotherapy.[24]

In the series described here, with these modifications, 17 of 21 (81%) patients reported normal ejaculation, with a mean seminal volume that did not differ significantly from that before lymphadenectomy. To date, in addition, four patients have fathered children. This series differs from that carried out before 1987, · in which a more extended lymphadenectomy was performed and ejaculation loss occurred in all patients.

With a mean follow-up of 28.9 months, 90.4% of patients are alive and free from disease, one patient has died of tumour and another patient has had a fatal heart attack while free from cancer. These data are in accord with the most recent reported series.

In the authors' opinion, greater nerve-sparing in patients with limited residual masses after chemotherapy, has enabled preservation of ejaculation to be achieved. This is an important issue in a group of young fertile patients.

References

1. Fossa S D, Ass N, Ous S et al. Histology of tumor residuals following chemotherapy in patients with advanced nonseminomatous testicular cancer. J Urol 1989; 142: 1239

2. Jaeger N, Weissbach L, Hartlapp J H, Vahlensieck W. Risk/benefit of treating retroperitoneal teratoid bulky tumors. Urology 1989; 34: 14

3. Peckham M J, Horwich A, Easton D F, Hendry W F. The management of advanced testicular teratoma. Br J Urol 1988; 62: 63

4. Vugrin D, Whitmore W F. The role of chemotherapy and surgery in the treatment of retroperitoneal metastases in advanced testis cancer. Cancer 1985; 55: 1874

5. Donohue J P, Rowland R G. Complications of retroperitoneal node dissection. J Urol 1981; 125: 338

6. Richie J R. Clinical stage 1 testicular cancer: the role of modified retroperitoneal lymphadenectomy. J Urol 1990; 144: 1160

7. Skinner D G, Melamud A, Lieskovsky G. Complications of thoracoabdominal retroperitoneal lymph node dissection. J Urol 1982; 127: 1107

8. Weissbach L, Boedefeld E A, Horstmann-Dubral B for the Testicular Tumor Study Group, Bonn. Surgical treatment of stage-I nonseminomatous germ cell testis tumor: final results of a prospective multicenter trial 1982–1987. Eur Urol 1990; 17: 97

9. Donohue J P. Retroperitoneal lymphadenectomy (RPLND) in low stage disease (staging RPLND) (one point of view). In: Khoury S, Küss R, Murphy G P, et al. Testicular cancer. New York: Liss, 1985; 203: 287–311

10. Fossa S D, Klepp O, Ous S et al. Unilateral retroperitoneal lymph node dissection in patients with nonseminomatous testicular tumor in clinical stage I. Eur Urol 1984; 10: 17

11. Lange P H, Chang W Y, Fraley E E. Fertility issues in the treatment of nonseminomatous testicular tumors. Urol Clin North Am 1987; 14: 731

12. Pizzocaro G, Salvoni R, Zanoni F. Unilateral lymphadenectomy in intraoperative stage I nonseminomatous germinal testis cancer. J Urol 1985; 134: 485

13. Colleselli K, Poisel S, Schachtner W, Bartsch G. Nerve-preserving bilateral lymphadenectomy: anatomical study and operative approach. J Urol 1990; 144: 293

14. Narayana P, Lange P H, Fraley E E. Ejaculation and fertility after extended retroperitoneal lymph node dissection for testicular cancer. J Urol 1982; 127: 685

15. Yaeger G H, Cowler A. Anatomical observations on the lumbar sympathetic nerve with evaluation of sympathectomies in organic vascular disease. Ann Surg 1948; 127: 953

16. Donohue J P, Foster R S, Rowland R G et al. Nerve-sparing retroperitoneal lymphadenectomy with preservation of ejaculation. J Urol 1990; 144: 287

17. Jewett M A, Kong Y P, Golberg S D et al. Retroperitoneal lymphadenectomy for testis tumor with nerve sparing for ejaculation. J Urol 1988; 139: 1220.

18. Fossa S D, Ous S, Abyholm T, Loeb M. Posttreatment fertility in patients with testicular cancer. Br J Urol 1985; 57: 204

19. Solè-Balcells F J, Villavicencio H, Germá J R, Algaba F. Effectiveness and morbidity of secondary retroperitoneal lymph node dissection after chemotherapy in testicular tumor. Eur Urol 1983; 9: 273.

20. Whitelaw G P, Smithwick R H. Some secondary effects of sympathectomy: with particular reference to disturbance of sexual function. N Engl J Med 1951; 245: 121

21. Donohue J P, Roth L M, Zachary J M et al. Cytoreductive surgery for metastatic testis cancer: tissue analysis of retroperitoneal masses after chemotherapy. J Urol 1982; 127: 1111

22. Donohue J P, Zachary J M, Maynard B R. Distribution of nodal metastases in nonseminomatous testis cancer. J Urol 1982; 128: 315

23. Weissbach L, Boedefeld E A for the Testicular Tumor Study Group. Localization of solitary and multiple metastases in stage II nonseminomatous testis tumor as basis for a modified staging lymph node dissection in stage I. J Urol 1987; 138: 77

24. Wood D P, Herr H W, Heller G et al. Distribution of retroperitoneal metastases after chemotherapy in patients with nonseminomatous germ cell tumors. J Urol 1992; 144: 1812

17

Lymph node surgery following chemotherapy for testis cancer

D. Kirk

Introduction

While discussion continues about the role of surgery in early stage non-seminomatous germ cell tumours (NSGCT),[1] its essential role after chemotherapy for bulky disease is uncontroversial.[2,3] However, opinions differ about the exact indications for, and about the timing of, surgery. The surgical approach and technique also raise issues. These are discussed in this chapter by reference to the author's personal surgical series, managed mainly in association with Professor Stanley Kaye of the Beatson Oncology Centre, Glasgow, UK. Of the 60 patients undergoing surgery since 1988, 58 had NSGCT, one seminoma and one paratesticular sarcoma. In tumour types other than NSGCT, surgery usually is palliative rather than curative. The discussion in this paper confines itself to the 58 patients with NSGCT.

Indications and strategies

Although low-volume retroperitoneal disease can be managed by primary surgical excision,[4] in extensive, bulky disease, surgery is used to excise residual disease remaining after platinum-based chemotherapy. Some authorities advocate surgical exploration in all patients even if post-treatment CT scans indicate complete resolution of the tumour mass,[5] a policy justified by the finding of viable tumour in a small proportion of patients. The author considers that this proportion is not large enough to justify what is an unnecessary operation in the majority, but careful follow-up is needed to identify the few patients who subsequently will develop disease requiring further treatment. Although, occasionally, it might be reasonable to observe a very small lesion after a clear response to chemotherapy, it is the author's usual practice to excise all residual tumours detectable on post-treatment CT scans. In selecting patients for surgery, it is important that good-quality CT scans are available. Careful comparision of scans before and after treatment is essential to avoid overlooking small-volume residual disease.

Elective surgery

Ideally, surgery follows completion of chemotherapy with normalization of tumour markers. When excision of residual disease reveals either well-differentiated tumour or a necrotic mass, cure can be confidently predicted.[3] Such elective surgery occurs in most of the author's patients but, occasionally, alternative strategies are required (Table 17.1).

Interventional surgery

Interventional surgery is used in patients with bulky disease that is not responding to chemotherapy.[6,7] It must be emphasized that this approach is applicable only to selected patients and it is *not* appropriate to operate on patients with active disease and raised markers if a response to chemotherapy is still occurring. However, in some patients despite aggressive chemotherapy, levels of markers will plateau or even start to rise. In this situation, excision of the tumour or at least aggressive debulking may help to bring the disease under control and allow subsequent chemotherapy to be effective (Fig. 17.1). Surgery must be timed to interfere as little as possible with the chemotherapy sequence, and the full course of chemotherapy must continue even after apparent complete excision of the tumour. In the author's hands (Table 17.2) this approach has been life-saving in some patients but in others results have been disappointing, emphasizing that very advanced NSGCT can still present an intractable problem. In two patients the abdominal para-aortic tumour accounted for the main bulk of the residual disease but

Strategy	No. of patients
Elective surgery	42*
Interventional surgery	6
Salvage surgery	10
Early relapse	5
Late relapse	4
Re operation	1

*Two patients have undergone second operations for thoracic, retrocrural and suprahilar recurrence — see text.

Table 17.1. Surgical strategies in 58 patients with NSGCT

151

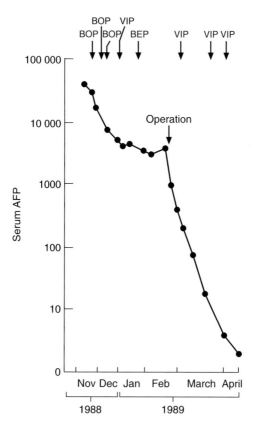

Figure 17.1. Example of effect of interventional surgery on tumour markers (serum alpha foetoprotein; AFP, kU/l) in patient with plateauing of markers on chemotherapy (BOP, cisplatin/vincristine/bleomycin; VIP, etoposide/ifosfamide/cisplatin; BEP, bleomycin/ etoposide/cisplatin). Note further chemotherapy starting promptly after surgery. Patient is alive and disease free at 5 years. (Reproduced from ref. 6 with permission of Editor of the British Journal of Cancer.)

Outcome	No. of patients
Alive and disease free	3
Alive, residual pelvic mass (6 years after surgery)	1
Died, active disease	1
Died chemotherapy complications	1

Table 17.2. Interventional surgery: outcome

proved to be necrotic, with active tumour in smaller-volume disease in the chest. In one of these patients (Fig. 17.2) the large (but necrotic) para-aortic tumour was excised with no effect on the level of tumour markers. In the other patient, surgery consisted of excision of the abdominal, retrocrural and all visible mediastinal disease, excision of the cervical nodes and left orchiectomy at a single operation. The para-aortic tumour, which formed the bulkiest mass, was necrotic. Active disease was present in the retrocrural area, mediastinum and in the cervical lymph nodes. Both these patients have died, the latter from his tumour, the other from complications of subsequent intensive chemotherapy. As stated above, interventional surgery is effective only in selected patients and probably will be most successful in disease confined to the abdomen. It can affect the outcome only if the bulk of the excised tissue consists of active tumour. If this is achieved, small volumes of tumour (for example in the lungs, as in one of the author's successfully treated patients) can be left until completion of chemotherapy.

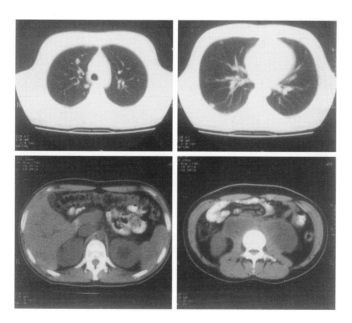

Figure 17.2. CT scans from patient with abdominal, retrocrural and pulmonary disease. Large para-aortic tumour contained necrotic tissue only. Retrocrural and pulmonary disease not excised. Subsequent death during intensive chemotherapy.

Salvage surgery

Salvage surgery is required where disease relapse occurs after apparent complete response, either early (within a few months of completion of chemotherapy) or after some years. Nine patients have undergone operation, having relapsed after previous treatment. Five relapses were early and four late (3–10 years), of whom one had had previous surgery. An additional patient with pelvic disease was referred after an incomplete operation plus radiotherapy in another centre. Further surgery removed the bulk of his disease, but a small amount of tumour remained infiltrating into the sidewall of the pelvis.

Patients who relapse early after chemotherapy probably still have active malignant teratoma and are best managed by surgery in combination with pre- and postoperative chemotherapy. One patient in whom this practice was not followed had a large tumour fungating through the posterior peritoneum and invading the serosa of several loops of small bowel (Fig. 17.3). Despite excision of the tumour with the involved, obstructed right kidney, he died with recurrent abdominal disease some months later.

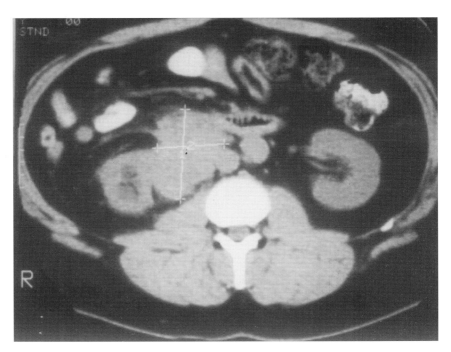

Figure 17.3. Early relapse after chemotherapy: large tumour invading serosa of small intestine. Note complete situs inversus.

Those who relapse several years after treatment are likely to have differentiated tumours and are best managed surgically. The four patients in this category have undergone surgery alone. One operation took place only recently. Three patients are alive and apparently disease free, 2 and 4 years after surgery without chemotherapy, although one patient's tumour contained mature adenocarcinoma for which he has refused further treatment.

The need for second operations after initial incomplete surgery is avoidable by ensuring that all these patients are treated in referral centres experienced in the medical and surgical management of the condition.

Surgical approach

Various incisions are described for abdominal lymph node excision.[8] The author excises most tumours through a full-length midline incision. If exposure is inadequate, extension in a 'Y' fashion by a left (usually) thoracoabdominal incision gives excellent access to the whole abdomen (Fig. 17.4), and readily allows mobilization of the left kidney, the spleen and pancreas, if necessary for suprahilar dissection, and access to the crural region. A modification of this approach, with an extra pleural lateral extension, has been described for routine use,[9] but most tumours are readily dealt with through the midline, and the thoracotomy when needed is well tolerated. The 'Y'-shaped wound heals without problem.

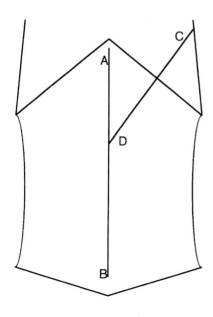

Figure 17.4. Standard initial midline incision (A–B) with thoracic extension (C–D) to improve access.

Thoracoabdominal extension in this way was necessary in five of these patients. A standard oblique thoracoabdominal incision was used in three more in whom a combined procedure with a thoracic surgical colleague was planned. However, it is often better to manage abdominal and thoracic disease at separate procedures.

Extent of operation

The author's practice is to excise completely the tumour visible on the CT scan, together with any other abnormal tissue present at operation, although the extent of the disease prior to chemotherapy is taken into account in planning the surgery. Some authors confine surgery to simple local excision of the residual mass;[3] others advocate a complete retroperitoneal clearance including full mobilization of the vena cava and aorta in all patients.[10] The author performs such surgery only when it is necessary to excise the tumour completely, as, in his opinion, the increased morbidity resulting from excision of normal tissue to achieve such a clearance is not justified. In his patients, relapses following surgery have been retrocrural, intrathoracic or, in one patient who also had a coincidental pulmonary recurrence, above the level of the renal arteries at the root of the superior mesenteric vessels. Two of these patients have undergone further surgery with curative intent and currently have no evidence of disease (Table 17.2). The third patient, who underwent surgery 1 year ago, has developed retrocrural disease, and is receiving chemotherapy. In none of the author's patients has relapse occurred in the area that would be cleared in a standard infrahilar dissection. What is essential is that excision is *complete* and extends into normal tissue. Careful examination of the whole retroperitoneum, with excision of any abnormal tissue distant from the main mass, is important and completeness of excision should be confirmed by margin biopsies. The author excises completely the testicular vessels on the side of the primary tumour with their surrounding fat down to the internal inguinal ring. In two patients, tumour nodules were present along the vessels, in both cases obviously visible at surgery. Although it is not the author's practice to send the margin biopsies routinely for frozen section, it is possible on frozen section to distinguish between active tumour and necrotic tissue. Obtaining confirmation by frozen section before extending the area of excision occasionally is appropriate, particularly when there is the possibility of invasion of the wall of one of the great vessels.

Outcome

Complete excision of tumour confined to the abdomen, however bulky and extensive, is normally possible (Table 17.3). In the author's limited experience with extensive pelvic disease, infiltration into the pelvic sidewall can be problematical. Intrathoracic disease is more difficult, partly because of the problem of ensuring that every one of multiple lung metastases has been excised, but also probably as a reflection of the inherent aggressiveness of disease which is this extensive at presentation. It is essential to have a close working relationship with a thoracic surgeon and to assess, in each patient, whether he is best served by combined surgery or by separate abdominal and thoracic procedures. In sequential operations, the author normally deals with the abdominal tumour first.

Histology (Table 17.4)
The presence of frankly malignant elements in excised tissue frequently necessitates further chemotherapy. Although necrotic tissue is reassuring as an indicator of the success of the chemotherapy, it does imply that surgery might have been unnecessary. The author's one postoperative death (due to bleomycin lung toxicity) followed a long and difficult operation. The CT size and appearance of the large tumour had not altered during chemotherapy, but it was completely necrotic. Tumour necrosis at one site, even if it is the main tumour mass, does not predict the state of tumour elsewhere.[11] In addition to the two patients in which this was encountered during interventional surgery, a patient who subsequently developed fatal pulmonary disease undetectable at the time of surgery had a completely necrotic abdominal tumour. Although it probably would be wise to excise bulky masses, even if known to be necrotic, the ability to distinguish necrotic from viable tumour would be of immense value in planning treatment in difficult situations.[12]

Disease site	Excision	
	Complete	Incomplete
Abdominal	56	0
Retrocrural	3	(1*)
Pelvic		2

*This patient underwent second operation for removal of recurrent retrocrural disease (plus lung and superior mediastinal recurence) and at present appears disease free.

Table 17.3. Outcome of surgery: excision rates

Histology	No. of patients
Differentiated teratoma	29
Malignant teratoma	9
Necrotic tissue	15*
Necrosis+ malignant teratoma	
(separate sites — see text)	2
Adenocarcinoma	2
Mixed differentiated teratoma/adenocarcinoma	1

*One patient subsequently developed fatal lung metastases

Table 17.4. Histology of excised tissue

Of the deaths occurring in the author's patients (Table 17.5), one, as described above, occurred from abdominal relapse after salvage surgery and might have been avoided with preoperative chemotherapy. That the remainder of the deaths occurred with thoracic disease or from chemotherapy-related toxicity indicates the important potential of abdominal surgery in this disease. However, one postoperative death resulting from bleomycin toxicity emphasizes that the problem these patients present transcends oncology and surgery, and experience in management of the condition by all involved, not least anaesthetist colleagues and intensive therapy unit staff, is essential.

In reporting the author's experience, tribute must be given to all those caring for the patients. Men with advanced NSGCT must be managed in referral centres, where close and regular communication between

Cause of death	No. of patients
Tumour related	
Abdominal	1
Thoracic	2
Chemotherapy related	
Renal failure	1
Bleomycin	1
(after-surgery)	

Table 17.5. Causes of death in non-survivors (5/58)

oncologist and surgeon is possible and where there is full backup from medical, nursing and other staff familiar with the problems presented by this disease and its treatment.

References

1. Ritchie J P. Editorial: Testis cancer — reduction in treatment morbidity with maintenance of treatment efficacy. J Urol 1994; 152: 431–432
2. Einhorn L H, Williams S D, Mandelbaum I, Donahue J. Surgical resection in disseminated testicular cancer following chemotherapeutic cytoreduction. Cancer 1981; 48: 904–908
3. Hendry W F, A'Hern R P, Hetherington H W et al. Para-aortic lymphadenectomy after chemotherapy for metastatic non seminomatous germ cell tumours: prognostic value and therapeutic benefit. Br J Urol 1993; 71: 208–213
4. De Bruin M J F M, Oesterhof G O N, Debruyne F M J. Nerve-sparing retroperitoneal lymphadenectomy for low stage testicular cancer. Br J Urol 1993; 71: 336–339
5. Wood D P Jr, Herr H W, Heller G et al. Distribution of retroperitoneal metastases after chemotherapy in patients with non-seminomatous germ cell tumours. J Urol 1992; 148: 1812–1816
6. Cassidy J, Lewis C R, Kaye S B, Kirk D. The changing role of surgery in metastatic non-seminomatous germ cell tumour. Br J Cancer 1992; 81: 127–129
7. Eastham J A, Wilson T G, Russell C et al. Surgical resection in patients with non-seminomatous germ cell tumour who fail to normalise serum tumour markers after chemotherapy. Urology 1994; 43: 74–80
8. Whitmore W F Jr, Morse M J. Surgery of testicular neoplasms. In: Walsh P C, Gittes R E, Perlmutter A D, Stamey T A (eds) Campbell's Urology, 5th ed. Philadelphia: Saunders, 1986: 2933-2954
9. Steiner M S, Nasland M J, Stutzman R E. A modified thoracoabdominal approach for retroperitoneal lymphadenectomy. J Urol 1993; 149: 23–25
10. Freiha F S, Shortliffe L D, Rouse R V et al. The extent of surgery after chemotherapy for advanced germ cell tumours. J Urol 1984; 132: 915–917
11. Gerl A, Clemm C, Schmeller N et al. Sequential resection of residual abdominal and thoracic masses after chemotherapy for metastatic non-seminomatous germ cell tumours. Br J Cancer 1994; 70: 960–965
12. Matsuyama H, Yamamoto N, Sakatoku J et al. Predictive values for the histologic nature of residual tumour mass after chemotherapy in patients with advanced testicular cancer. Urology 1994; 44: 392–399.

Index